Letting Go
of Perfect

Letting Go of Perfect

A GAY MAN'S GUIDE TO HEALING FROM BODY DYSMORPHIA

DANIEL O'SHAUGHNESSY

Foreword by Dr Miguel Toribio-Mateas

Jessica Kingsley Publishers
London and Philadelphia

First published in Great Britain in 2026 by Jessica Kingsley Publishers
An imprint of John Murray Press

1

Copyright © Daniel O'Shaughnessy 2026
Foreword © Dr Miguel Toribio-Mateas 2026

The information contained in this book is not intended to replace the services
of trained medical professionals or to be a substitute for medical advice. You
are advised to consult a doctor on any matters relating to your health, and in
particular on any matters that may require diagnosis or medical attention.

Content Warning: This book mentions bullying; drugs; eating disorders;
homophobia; self-harm; sexual trauma; suicidal thoughts; trauma.

A CIP catalogue record for this title is available from the
British Library and the Library of Congress

ISBN 978 1 80501 798 1
eISBN 978 1 80501 799 8

Printed and bound in Great Britain by Clays Ltd

Jessica Kingsley Publishers' policy is to use papers that are natural,
renewable and recyclable products and made from wood grown in
sustainable forests. The logging and manufacturing processes are expected
to conform to the environmental regulations of the country of origin.

Jessica Kingsley Publishers
Carmelite House
50 Victoria Embankment
London EC4Y 0DZ

www.jkp.com

John Murray Press
Part of Hodder & Stoughton Ltd
An Hachette Company

The authorised representative in the EEA is Hachette Ireland,
8 Castlecourt Centre, Dublin 15, D15 XTP3, Ireland (email: info@hbgi.ie)

To the ones who stand with you,
unwavering, as you navigate the messy
and beautiful process of healing.

Those are your people.

Contents

Exercises

Preface

WELCOME TO A JOURNEY THAT IS RAW, unfiltered, and unapolo-
getically real. This book is a cocktail of my lived experiences,
professional expertize, healing, and academic knowledge that I've
woven together to offer something honest and true. It's a reflection
of my path, one filled with trials, tribulations, breakthroughs, and setbacks, written in the hope that it serves as a guide and companion for
you as you navigate your own journey of healing.

If you're holding this book, it likely means that body dysmorphia
or insecurities about your body have touched your life in some way.
Whether you've experienced it personally or know someone who has,
this isn't an easy topic to face head-on. But I want to assure you: this
book doesn't shy away from the uncomfortable. It's not dressed up in
fluffy language. It's raw, to the point, and steeped in the reality of what
it means to heal – especially when you're part of the gay community,
where the pressure to conform to specific body ideals can feel relentless.

In these pages, I've reflected on my own healing journey, shared personal stories, and combined my professional experience as a nutritionist
with my master's degree, which focused on the integration of mental
health and lived experience, to offer insights, guidance, and hope. You'll
find a blend of academic analysis, practical strategies, and emotional
vulnerability. This book is not just a resource – it's a conversation, one
that invites you to reflect, to question, and to nurture your own healing.

I'm not here to promise you that healing will be a straight path
or an easy one. It's messy, painful, and often feels like you're digging
up things you thought were long buried. But as you move forward,
you'll uncover the strength, wisdom, and resilience that have always
been inside you. In the coming chapters, you'll find an exploration of

body dysmorphia, how nutrition impacts our mental health, the role of trauma, and much more. Each chapter will guide you through practical strategies, personal insights, and exercises designed to help you heal your relationship with your body and mind. You'll learn to rewrite the narrative that body dysmorphia has tried to impose on you and reclaim a sense of self that is grounded in compassion and self-love.

This book isn't just about finding peace with your reflection – it's about finding peace with who you are. And yes, it's going to be uncomfortable at times. But discomfort is part of growth, and on the other side of that discomfort is a version of you that is more empowered, more self-assured, and more at peace than ever before.

What sets this book apart are the exercises woven throughout its chapters. They are designed to help you dismantle the thought patterns that keep you trapped in cycles of self-criticism, challenge your internal narrative, and develop a new, compassionate relationship with your body and mind. Each exercise has been created with the intention of offering you tangible steps towards self-love, growth, and mental wellness.

And I mean, *really* take the time to do the exercises. If you're like me, it's easy to skip over them when reading self-help books, but these moments of reflection are where the real work begins. Allow yourself to pause, reflect, and revisit as much as you need to. The goal is to support you in shifting your mindset and to help you create lasting change. This is your journey, and there's no right or wrong way to walk it.

Finally, I want you to know that you're not alone in this process. Healing is not something you do in isolation – it's something we walk through together, with a community of support, understanding, and acceptance. While this book is intended to offer guidance and hope, it's not a substitute for therapy or professional support. If you feel overwhelmed or believe you would benefit from additional help, I strongly encourage you to seek support from a qualified therapist or healthcare professional. Reaching out for support is a powerful step towards self-acceptance and growth. I invite you to stay connected – to yourself, to the practices of self-love, and to the community we're building together. We all deserve love, respect, and acceptance, exactly as we are.

I look forward to walking alongside you.

Daniel ♥

Foreword

THERE ARE MOMENTS IN LIFE when you witness someone step into the fullness of who they are, not just despite their struggles but because of them. This book – raw, unfiltered, and achingly honest – is the result of one such transformation.

I met Daniel in 2010, which now feels almost like a previous life. Even then, there was an intensity to his curiosity, a hunger – not just for knowledge but for something deeper. Over the years, I watched him wrestle with the complexities of body image, self-worth, and the unrelenting pressure of societal ideals. But more than that, I watched him do the work. The deep, uncomfortable, necessary work of self-acceptance.

This book is the supporting evidence of that journey.

For many of us, particularly those of us in the LGBTQ+ community, body dysmorphia is more than an abstract concept. It is a daily reality, shaped by cultural expectations, childhood narratives, and the often unspoken belief that our worth is measured by how closely we align with a prescribed ideal. I know this struggle intimately. The shame, the self-doubt, the endless striving for a version of 'perfection' always remains just out of reach, no matter how much you hit the gym or how much Botox you have. And I know the toll it takes.

But I also know what lies beyond it.

Daniel has beautifully woven together personal experience, clinical expertise, and deep compassion to create an exquisite guide that doesn't just inform – it heals. This is not a book that offers quick fixes or surface-level solutions. It is an invitation: to question, to reflect, to challenge the narratives we've been given, and, ultimately, to let go of what no longer serves us. It is about reclaiming our right to inhabit our bodies with kindness rather than criticism, with curiosity rather than control.

What sets this book apart is its intersection of science and lived experience. It is both a map and a mirror. A map that provides the tools and insights necessary for navigating the complexities of body dysmorphia, and a mirror that reflects back the truth that you are not alone in this. That healing is possible. That self-acceptance is not a luxury but a birthright.

But let me tell you: this journey is not linear. And I say that with love because I have been there myself. In fact, I am still there, because the work is ongoing. There will be days when old patterns creep back in, when the voice of self-criticism echoes loudly, convincing you that slipping into self-sabotage is the only way to cope with the unsettling familiarity of past habits; as if, in a single moment, all your progress had unravelled. But there will also be moments of clarity, of peace, of joy in the sheer beauty of being present in the here and now, without expectations. Hold on to those moments and intentionally cultivate that awareness, trusting that they will multiply.

Daniel, thank you for writing the book so many of us needed but didn't know how to ask for. Thank you for your vulnerability, your wisdom, and your refusal to sugarcoat the truth. And to the reader: may these pages serve as a guide, a companion, and a reminder that your worth was never meant to be measured in numbers or comparisons – whether with the image in the mirror or with anyone else. You are, and always have been, enough.

With deep admiration and gratitude,

Dr Miguel Toribio-Mateas
Clinical Neuroscientist and Honorary Research Fellow
at Cardiff University's School of Psychology

CHAPTER 1

My Story

SHALL WE START BY SAYING WHAT WE DON'T LIKE ABOUT OURSELVES? Don't worry, I'll go first. I don't like that my hairline is receding; I feel I'm carrying too much fat around the middle; my skin flares easily, particularly when I'm stressed or eat foods that I know I'm sensitive to; and I feel so uncomfortable in my body when I haven't exercised – sluggish, unmotivated, and out of sync with myself. I hate looking at my reflection but love to criticize it and constantly seek ways to improve it. I'm also a great saboteur. When I'm on a health kick, I get these little voices in my head telling me to binge on foods high in sugar and fat: 'Don't worry, you deserve a treat – the diet can start on Monday.' These foods offer temporary relief from life stressors, allowing me to live comfortably numb in a bubble, but in the end, they always make me feel worse. I then beat myself up about breaking my diet, adding to the feelings of inadequacy when I look in the mirror.

I've felt like this for as long as I can remember, my head plagued with self-criticism that never quietens, acting as background noise – waiting for the right moment to surface when I catch my reflection or feel my clothes are a bit too tight. These thoughts are a constant hum in the back of my mind, critiquing every aspect of my appearance and behaviour, never relenting for a moment to let me catch my breath, and following me to work, parties, and even relationships. It's been a long journey to be able to share these feelings of inadequacy with others. Whenever I tried, the typical response was, 'Don't be silly – you look great,' or something similar. To avoid burdening others and enduring these predictable reactions, I kept it secret for a long time.

However, everything changed when I decided to take a chance and be vulnerable, sharing the inner workings of my mind with the world.

The day I decided to open up about what I'd been hiding for years felt like stepping off a cliff. I was terrified of judgement, but I couldn't carry the weight of it any more. I needed to be heard. This courageous step marked the beginning of my healing journey, changed my worldview, and redefined my professional approach as a nutritionist.

I'm the loud complainer in the silent battle that many of us face – the battle with body dysmorphia. I used to think people might dismiss me, or worse, pity me. But instead I found connection. The more I shared, the more I realized how many others were quietly fighting the same battle.

As a nutritionist, the journey to this point hasn't been straightforward. Over the past decade, I have advised others on optimal diets and health strategies, testing every conceivable nutritional plan myself – from meticulously counting calories to eliminating entire food groups. I prided myself on my disciplined approach to health, believing that a balanced diet and rigorous exercise regimen, paired with effective stress management, comprised the key to wellness.

Despite my professional expertize, I found myself grappling with a personal health crisis, which challenged everything I knew about health and wellness. What I once deemed a foolproof formula for physical health barely scratched the surface of true well-being. The strict routines and dietary restrictions I embraced were merely superficial solutions – Band-Aids that temporarily covered, but ultimately could not heal, the deeper pain lurking beneath. I was full to the brim, weighed down by unresolved trauma and a deep-seated shame about my sexuality. I was completely unaware of how this was manifesting, but an incessant feeling of inadequacy, especially about my body, accompanied me daily. Looking in the mirror, I thought it was normal to critique every inch of my body with thoughts that I was too fat or that my arms weren't big enough and had to be bigger. It would not be worth it for my anxiety if I didn't do a rigorous workout at least five times per week; missing a session was met with dread, which ironically would spawn a cascade of binge eating. This only deepened my loathing for my reflection. I lived under the illusion that this was normal and that such struggles were just part of being a gay man, especially when comparing myself to others on the dance floor at the weekend or trying to get my body ready for the next big gay party or beach-ready for Mykonos. There was always something to improve, always a way in which I fell short. Unbeknownst to me at the time, I was battling body dysmorphia – a reality far from normal and far from healthy.

Admitting I needed to heal was the hardest part, but I am proud to say that I have embarked on a lifelong journey of healing, broadening my awareness and dedicating the necessary time to truly confront and commit to mending my wounds. Today, I write with the hope of offering visibility and vulnerability to those who may find themselves in a similar position. This isn't just another topic; it's a deeply personal journey that I'm unveiling, and my utmost goal is to present it with genuine authenticity.

It is important to note that the path to healing is continuous; this book is not a declaration of victory over body dysmorphia or a proclamation that my life is now flawless. Rather, my aim is for it to serve as a road map for other gay individuals who are navigating similar challenges, providing guidance from my lessons learnt and perhaps a measure of solace as they too embark on their own paths to healing.

Maybe you're here because you're ready to start healing too or maybe you're just curious. Wherever you are, know that healing is possible – and it doesn't have to be perfect.

Early years

I grew up immersed in the early 1990s diet culture, where 'diet' labels were synonymous with health. As a child of just ten years old, my days were dominated by diet cola and the latest fad diets plastered across every TV screen and magazine. My mother, a diet consultant for a popular weight loss brand, filled our home with diet foods, magazines, and endless discussions about the best ways to shed a few pounds. It became commonplace to hear about the perpetual cycle of dieting from those around me – constant talk of body improvement, followed by the inevitable 'falling off the waggon' and declarations of 'I'll start again on Monday' or 'It's treat day today', at their weekly weigh-ins as they stripped down to their underwear in an effort to weigh a pound or two less. While this could have laid the foundations for my career as a nutritionist, it also ingrained a belief in the normalcy and necessity of yo-yo dieting.

My adolescence brought its own challenges. I was a late bloomer, overweight, gay, and ginger – attributes that made me the target of relentless bullying. The taunts of 'fat, ginger faggot' haunted my walks through the school corridors, where I tried desperately to remain invisible. Discovering the gym was a revelation – a sanctuary where I could attempt to build physical and psychological armour against the abuse and do this alone without the fear of being picked last for the football team again.

Leaving school marked a significant turning point. My early adult years brought new freedoms but also new battles. I gradually lost weight and began to carve out an identity separate from the bullied child reflected back at me in the mirror. However, the criticisms I grew up with still echoed around me, especially as I ventured onto the gay scene. It was there that my body dysmorphia truly stepped into the limelight, though I was wholly unconscious of it at the time.

My life became a regimented cycle: weekends on the gay scene and weekday nights striving in the gym for two hours after work. My focus was unyielding – build bigger muscles, reduce fat, and maximize protein intake. In the gym, I watched the bodybuilders with a mixture of admiration and envy, yearning to join the ranks of those who confidently flaunted their physiques, tops off, in the clubs. These men appeared to belong to an exclusive club, bonded by their impressive chests and arms, which only fuelled my self-doubt and deepened my resolve to achieve a similar form. As I pushed myself harder, I began to realize that this wasn't just about achieving a body that looked right; it was about overcoming the feelings of inadequacy that haunted me at each reflection in the mirror.

Anabolic steroids

As my friends delved into the world of anabolic steroids, I found myself increasingly caught up in their discussions about various stacks – the combinations of steroids they were using – and how they managed the side effects. Enquiries about other gymgoers I admired were often dismissed with a casual, 'He's on gear.'

Following a turbulent breakup, and in an effort to start anew at 32 years old, I saw steroids as my only avenue to boost self-esteem

– superficially, a mix of slight revenge on my ex and the determination to 'get someone better' but mainly seeing them as the only path to finally feeling good about myself. A quick message to a friend soon connected me with a steroid dealer, who advised over text on suitable options for beginners and arranged a meeting the next day. That meeting marked the beginning of my continuous four-year cycle on anabolic steroids.

I harboured a little secret again, and it gave me a thrill, almost akin to the buzz I sometimes felt hiding my sexuality when I was younger. Not only did the scales start to tip in the right direction, but I also experienced a surge of energy and the beginnings of a new-found, albeit hollow, confidence that others noticed. I lifted heavier weights in the gym, indulged my appetite with my ramped-up metabolism, and most importantly, I started to attract attention from the 'it' crowd I had once admired at the gym and in clubs. Initially, this attention was shocking, but my ego soon swelled in tandem with my muscles. I shrugged off comments from friends and family about my rapid muscle gain, claiming it was all due to hard training and a good diet.

I thought I had sidestepped the side effects. I didn't experience the typical 'roid rage' often associated with anabolic steroids, so I assumed I was in the clear. However, routine blood tests revealed elevated liver enzymes and raised cholesterol levels – common side effects of steroids. I convinced myself that milk thistle, a herb known to support liver function, and fish oil for heart health would mitigate these issues. Yet the side effects gradually worsened and my body was starting to break down. My muscles became so tight that walking 100 metres from my house required stops to catch my breath and stretch. Nights were restless; I would wake at 2 a.m. after just a few hours of sleep needing to eat something to return to sleep. Then, balding at the crown of my head began, another common side effect, prompting me to start using hair loss medication and later undergo a hair transplant.

Every time I discussed these side effects with others, they suggested another pill to counteract them. I felt like a walking pharmacy, yet I was content to deceive myself into believing I was taking good care of my health, even as I took stronger steroids with each visit to the dealer. Typically, steroid cycles last for about eight weeks before a break to allow natural testosterone production to recover. This was not an option for me; my ego couldn't face what would surface if I stopped, so I continued using steroids consistently for over four years, occasionally lowering the dose to give the illusion of recovery and playing buckaroo with side-effect medication as and when I needed to.

What I didn't anticipate were the severe mental health side effects that crept in subtly. It wasn't just manageable anxiety that I could try to alleviate with a magnesium pill or two. I became hypersensitive to stress, neurotic in my dating life – particularly with rejection, and breathless even at the sound of an email pinging on my laptop. The superficial Band-Aid of self-esteem began to peel away. My body dysmorphia didn't just return; it intensified. The reflection in the mirror didn't match how others saw me, and thoughts of self-criticism and the need for improvement resurfaced. My response was to take longer and heavier steroid cycles, train harder, and eat more. All this was an attempt to feel more comfortable in my skin and seek validation on the dance floor during weekend parties, oblivious – or perhaps unwilling to acknowledge – the increasing strain I was placing on my body.

The professional paradox

The irony of it all was that I appeared as serene as a swan gliding down the river, even though beneath the surface I was frantically swimming against the current. The bullying trauma I endured and having to hide my sexuality had ingrained a belief in me that I needed to hide any struggle. I had chosen a career as a nutritionist, a role that often seemed to epitomize perfectionism in every aspect. There is a deep cultural expectation that nutritionists and fitness professionals lead perfectly healthy lives, and I felt this very burden. There I was, smiling with a kale smoothie in an Instagram photo, praising its health benefits, just moments after taking a steroid injection. I'm not going to lie; deep down there were ripples of cognitive dissonance, but like with my shame and everything else, I just filed it away or convinced myself I was doing the right thing.

What the public saw was just one of the many masks I donned. I had a drawer full of masks, and I pulled them out as easily as I needed to. I knew deep down this wasn't my authentic self, but this is what I felt I had to do to succeed, to be taken seriously. It's what everyone does professionally; you don't show vulnerability because it's awkward and not luxury, I was even told.

While I love being a nutritionist, the role has paradoxically brought out parts of my shadow self and sometimes exacerbated my body dysmorphia. Experimenting with the latest fasting trends or adopting a ketogenic diet by eliminating carbohydrates from my meal plan were just some of the controls I imposed on myself. These restrictions were a means to both improve, control, and unconsciously punish myself. Given that people frequently sought my advice on diets and lifestyles, their expectations served as a subtle encouragement to further tighten these restrictions and refine my approach. Whenever I chose a food option that is generally considered unhealthy, people would often remark, 'Oh, I thought you were a nutritionist,' which would plunge me further into shame, adding another layer of complexity to my body dysmorphia.

The need for healing

My journey was both physically gruelling and emotionally revealing, laying the groundwork for personal and professional growth that went far beyond the gym. Through this process, I came to understand the true extent of my body dysmorphia and the mental transformation required to truly heal. Each session in the gym, and every comparison to others, was a step not just towards a stronger body but towards a deeper self-awareness and eventual acceptance of my own unique journey.

I had reached a point where criticizing my body became a routine, emotionless activity every time I looked in the mirror, and oddly, it was something I was almost content to engage in. I was trapped in a relentless cycle of bulking and cutting – a regimen well-known among bodybuilders, where phases of muscle growth are interspersed with periods of reducing body fat by reducing calories. Despite the clear signs of distress, I didn't consider myself to have an eating disorder like bulimia or anorexia, which I viewed as more extreme conditions, so I saw no reason to consult my doctor regarding body dysmorphia. While I was aware of my tendencies to binge eat and impose strict dietary restrictions on myself, these behaviours seemed common among my colleagues and others within the gay scene, which normalized my experiences and further obscured the seriousness of my condition.

My life was crumbling around me; my professional life was highly stressful; I was entangled in a family dispute; I jumped from one unhealthy relationship to another; and I was partying too much. The irony around partying was that my consciousness was geared towards living my best life among my 'chosen family'. For me, it was a combination of a chance to numb myself from the hell I was going through and a desperate attempt to seek validation from others, hoping to feel just 1 per cent better about myself than the routine misery I put myself through.

I had ignored or blocked out the well-documented mental health side effects associated with anabolic steroids. I didn't think I had depression as I was highly functional. Yes, I was anxious and in therapy but being anxious felt normal to me, and I had accepted it as part of who I was. However, I began experiencing increasingly intense, dark thoughts about ending my life, signalling a severe problem. This was a critical wake-up call for me, adding yet more complexity to my situation. It's strange; you want help, but the fuss of the vulnerability step is so overwhelmingly difficult. For me, I couldn't bear the thought of bathing in shame, acknowledging my failures, having to take off the masks I wore daily, and having to admit my use of anabolic steroids and my struggle with body dysmorphia. Looking back, I see this was not the best approach, and there were many resources available where I could have sought help.

Gradually, I came to the stark realization that my relentless pursuit of physical perfection was overshadowing my mental well-being. Each day became a mirror of the last, where the focus was solely on my appearance, ignoring the psychological toll it was taking. The façade of control I maintained through my diet and fitness regime began to crack, revealing the mental strain hidden beneath. This shift in perspective was alarming yet necessary, as it highlighted how intertwined my mental health was with my physical practices. It became clear that if I were to truly heal, I needed to address not just the physical symptoms but also the root of my psychological distress. This acknowledgement marked the beginning of my journey towards seeking deeper, more holistic forms of healing.

Turning points

Entering therapy was one of the best decisions I've ever made. It not only helped me reframe my thoughts but also feel more present in my body, rather than constantly feeling like an anxious wreck. The journey hasn't been straightforward; it involved setting boundaries, embracing vulnerability, and being truthful with both myself and my therapist. This didn't happen all at once; even now, I struggle with trust and fully letting go in a therapeutic setting.

However, it was ayahuasca (a plant-based psychedelic medicine from the Amazon) and psilocybin (the active compound in magic mushrooms) that truly enabled me to achieve a transformative understanding of myself. My curiosity about these substances was piqued by documentaries and books and how psychedelics were gaining traction as a mental health treatment (Nutt, Spriggs, and Erritzoe, 2023), prompting a decision that was far from easy. I recall how terrified I was initially – hesitating when a friend suggested a psychedelic retreat might be beneficial. My immediate reaction was, 'But I may cry,' which stopped me in my tracks and motivated me to book a space on a retreat. These therapies aren't accessible in the UK due to legal restrictions, leading me to travel to places where participating in such ceremonies is legal and supervised under the guidance of a shaman.

Psychedelic therapy is intense and certainly not for everyone. For me, it was exactly what I needed – a challenging confrontation with my ego that transformed my perceptions and self-assumptions. It was a journey of forgiveness – not just towards others but primarily towards myself – and marked the beginning of a genuine commitment to personal healing. This process allowed me to release years of accumulated anger, trauma, and pain. It provided me with a fresh perspective on my body, fostering a desire to respect it and reducing my dependency on external validation. Consequently, I stopped using steroids, which I had relied on to maintain a cycle of self-competition and feelings of inadequacy. Now, I visit the gym and eat with my health in mind, not just to gain muscle mass while enduring numerous side effects. I've learnt to manage my triggers, no longer obsessing over calorie or protein intake; I naturally eat well without extremes and don't think too much about skipping the gym, especially if I am tired. Looking in the mirror, I might not see the most muscular version of myself, but I've never felt more at peace with who I am. These behaviours didn't happen all at once. Gradually, over time and with self-compassion, they were implemented bit by bit.

It's important to note that psychedelics aren't a magic bullet. While they've had a profound impact on me, they are just one of many ways to begin seeing the path forward. Healing is deeply personal, and what works for one person may not resonate with another. Psychedelics simply illuminate potential paths; the real work begins afterwards. This involves ongoing therapy or other forms of support to help process and integrate the insights gained, as well as a personal commitment to making meaningful changes.

You cannot attain perfection, and there is beauty in that. Accept yourself as you are, flaws and all, and make an effort to not let passing thoughts ensnare you. There are still days when I don't feel good about myself and get triggered, but I have learnt practices that help me not become overly attached to these thoughts or to explore the root causes of my reactions to them. This becomes easier with practice, which I will discuss later in this book.

Professionally, these experiences have reshaped my understanding of health, enriching how I work with clients and broadening my perspective on what constitutes true health. To structure these insights, I completed a master's programme in transdisciplinary practice (a professional practice MSc), focusing my research on psychedelics, mental health, and lived experience. This has enabled me to create a framework with academic rigour that integrates the lessons from psychedelics, facilitating mindset changes that support the journey to self-love and holistic health.

This book's purpose

The purpose of this book is to bring attention to an often unspoken issue in the gay community: the lived experiences of those struggling with body dysmorphia.

This book goes beyond sharing lessons from my personal journey. It merges my background in nutrition and academia to provide a practical guide with actionable steps aimed at cultivating a more compassionate relationship with yourself and celebrating your uniqueness and life experiences.

In this book, we will explore the essential relationship between nutrition, mindset, and self-compassion, which collectively underpin holistic health. This integration is crucial for anyone looking to heal their relationship with their body and navigate the complex challenges of body dysmorphia. Good nutrition is fundamental, but it must be balanced and not overly prescriptive to truly fuel the body and support the right mindset. Without this balance, even the most scientifically sound diets can fail.

Central to overcoming body dysmorphia is transforming one's mindset, a theme that permeates this journey. It involves reconstructing harmful thought patterns and beliefs about oneself and developing more positive, affirming mental frameworks. This healthy mindset underpins sustainable eating patterns and habits, aids in understanding setbacks, and supports lasting changes that go beyond mere health to thriving.

Equally important is nurturing a compassionate inner dialogue. Struggles should be met with acceptance and kindness rather than criticism, facilitating a recovery rooted in understanding and patience rather than discipline alone. Together, these elements not only address the symptoms of body dysmorphia but also empower individuals to lead healthier, more fulfilled lives.

This book is structured into sections that progressively tackle the multifaceted nature of body dysmorphia, starting with an exploration of its roots and impacts, particularly within the gay community. Subsequent chapters explore practical strategies for nutrition and mental health, enriched with personal anecdotes to provide a relatable and empathetic perspective.

Letting Go of Perfect: A Gay Man's Guide to Healing from Body Dysmorphia is not merely informative – it acts as a companion for gay men on their path to healing from body dysmorphia, offering hope and affirming the strength found in self-acceptance. It is a call to embrace one's journey towards a loving relationship with their own reflection, paving the way for a life free from the shadows of dysmorphia to one filled with freedom, authenticity, and pride.

Building on this foundation, by sharing my own journey and those of others within the gay community, this book aims to create a bond of solidarity and support. I hope to inspire not just understanding and hope but also a collective strength in vulnerability, encouraging you to face your deepest fears and insecurities with openness and courage.

While this book primarily focuses on the experiences of gay men navigating body dysmorphia, I recognize that body image issues and dysmorphia affect individuals across the entire queer spectrum – bisexual, non-binary, and trans people included. Each identity faces unique pressures and challenges, particularly where gender presentation, attraction, and societal expectations intersect. My hope is that while this book is anchored in my lived experience as a gay man, many queer readers will find insights that resonate with their own journeys towards self-acceptance.

Exercise: Your current relationship with your body

Before we begin, I'd like to invite you to pause and reflect on the relationship you have with your body. It may be useful to keep a journal handy as we explore various themes in this book. I encourage you to just take a pen and write without thinking too much; just let the ink flow onto the paper. This process of spontaneous writing can help uncover deeper insights and emotions. Whether it's your thoughts, feelings, anger, disagreements, or revelations, jot them down as they come to you throughout this book.

1. Can you identify a moment or event that significantly shaped your thoughts around your body image?
2. What are your nutrition and lifestyle like? What's good about it, and what could be improved?
3. How has your relationship with your body changed over the years?
4. What are the most persistent negative thoughts you have about your body, and where do you think they come from?
5. How do you react to compliments or criticism about your appearance?
6. In what ways do societal or cultural standards of beauty influence your feelings about your body?
7. What practices or habits have you found helpful in nurturing a healthier body image?
8. How do your feelings about your body impact your relationships and social interactions?
9. What does self-care look like to you, and how does it relate to your body image?
10. Are there aspects of your body or appearance that you've learnt to appreciate more over time?

These questions are designed to guide you through a personal exploration of how you perceive your physical self and the factors influencing this perception. Reflecting on these questions can help you better understand the journey you are on towards self-acceptance and body positivity.

CHAPTER 2

Introduction to Body Dysmorphia: Beyond the Surface

W E LIVE IN A WORLD DOMINATED BY MEDIA, where we relent-lessly consume content 24/7. We are constantly flooded with images of what 'perfect' looks like, and it's easy to get caught up in this, triggering comparisons and making us believe that we're falling short. Emerging from this landscape is body dysmorphia, a condition widely misunderstood and cloaked in stigma. Far from being merely about physical appearance, body dysmorphia is a complex psychological condition. It traps people in endless cycles of obsessive thoughts and behaviours, rooted deeply in the psyche. It stems from a variety of underlying causes and is often hidden, both from those experiencing it and the people around them. The path to recognition and recovery is frequently complicated for those with body dysmorphia because they are unaware of how much control it has over their lives.

Body dysmorphia, or body dysmorphic disorder (BDD), is when someone becomes fixated on what they perceive as flaws in their appearance – flaws that others often don't even notice. This can cause significant stress for the person affected and impact their ability to function normally in everyday life. According to the National Health Service (NHS 2023), the symptoms of BDD include:

- Persistent worry about a particular body area (which is usually the face).

- Often comparing looks to others.
- Frequent use of mirrors or avoiding mirrors altogether.
- Endless effort to conceal perceived flaws.
- Skin picking.

Body dysmorphia can feel like being stuck in an endless loop. One negative thought leads to another, and before you know it, you're spiralling (see Figure 2.1). These thoughts, such as 'I'm not good enough' or 'I don't look right', often lead to self-scrutiny, where someone fixates on perceived flaws in their appearance and how they can change it. This scrutiny manifests in behaviours like constantly checking mirrors, comparing themselves to others, or even avoiding social situations altogether. These actions only serve to reinforce low self-esteem and worsen mental health, which brings them back to the same negative thoughts, thus perpetuating the cycle.

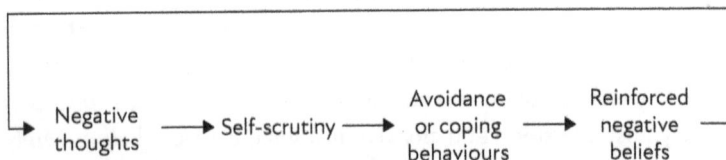

Negative thoughts ⟶ Self-scrutiny ⟶ Avoidance or coping behaviours ⟶ Reinforced negative beliefs

Figure 2.1. *Imagine a thought like 'I'm not good enough' popping into your mind. From there, you might start picking apart every detail of your appearance, leading you to avoid people, mirrors, or events. It's exhausting, and it feeds right back into more negative thoughts.*

Body dysmorphia goes far deeper than simply disliking your reflection. For me, it wasn't just about disliking what I saw in the mirror. It was the constant feeling that I wasn't enough – that no matter how much I changed, I'd still be stuck with the same broken version of myself. It's an ongoing battle with how you see yourself, tied to emotions and mental health in ways that are difficult to understand. It extends beyond surface-level dissatisfaction to a deep and enduring sense of self-rejection that no amount of physical alteration can cure. This mental struggle becomes ingrained in your self-perception, often tied to complex psychological issues that significantly affect your overall well-being.

Body dysmorphia: a drastic term for a hidden struggle

When people hear the term 'body dysmorphia', it can sound quite drastic – something extreme and far removed from everyday experience. What's even harder is that body dysmorphia often hides in plain sight. It's easy to put on a brave face and laugh in front of others while quietly battling these thoughts alone. It's not always about visible actions like avoiding mirrors, overexercising, or undergoing cosmetic treatments; sometimes it shows up in more familiar ways, like second-guessing your appearance before leaving the house or feeling unsettled in a room full of people. It's that nagging inner voice saying you're not good enough, even if others don't see what you're obsessing over.

Body dysmorphia exists on a spectrum. For some, it's subtle and lingering; for others, it's all-consuming. But it always comes from the same place – feeling like your appearance somehow falls short. And while the term might sound severe, many of us have unknowingly encountered these feelings at different times. Body dysmorphia isn't something that only happens to a few people – it's a hidden struggle that so many face. You might know someone battling it, even if they've never said a word.

The aim of this chapter is to examine the varied nature of body dysmorphia beyond a superficial understanding. We will look at its psychological roots, its specific impact on the gay community, and address the widespread misunderstandings and stigmas associated with it. Through this chapter, I hope to not only deepen your understanding of body dysmorphia but also inspire more empathy. I want to challenge the prejudices we don't always recognize and learn how we can support both ourselves and others who are navigating this silent battle.

What causes body dysmorphia?

Body dysmorphia isn't something that just happens. It's the result of many things coming together – genetics, environment, and the world around us – that together shape how someone sees their body. These influences interact in ways that are unique to each person, making the condition as individual as the person experiencing it. Let's take a closer look at the primary contributors behind body dysmorphia.

Genetic

Genetic factors play a role, with research suggesting that some of us are wired to be more susceptible to body dysmorphia due to variations in brain structure and the function of chemical messengers in the brain known as neurotransmitters (Weiffenbach and Kundu 2015). BDD also shares similarities with obsessive-compulsive disorder with regard to a heightened focus on minute details, particularly regarding one's appearance (Tasios and Michopoulos 2017).

Environmental

Our environment, especially in our early years, shapes how we see ourselves. For example, as was partly my case, growing up in a family where there is a focus on appearance or dieting can plant seeds of insecurity that grow over time. It's also not just what is said directly to us, but the subtle cues we pick up about how much our worth seems tied to how we look. These cues often shape our self-perception unconsciously. In some cases, children mirror the behaviours they see, absorbing the body-related anxieties of those around them. In environments where weight or appearance is a frequent topic of discussion, the risk of developing body dysmorphia becomes much higher.

Workplaces and social settings can all influence how we see ourselves. In competitive environments, where physical appearance is linked to performance – such as in sports, dance, or the fashion industry – the pressure to meet a certain standard is relentless. The constant comparison with others can fuel perfectionism, and before long, you're not just chasing excellence – you're obsessing over every perceived flaw. Even in less obvious settings like corporate environments, appearance can be tied to job opportunities or promotions, reinforcing the belief that looking a certain way is essential for success.

But it's not just these competitive spaces; everyday social settings also shape our self-image. The subtle judgements and societal expectations encountered in schools or among peers can significantly impact how we view ourselves. For many, these pressures are compounded by more overt forms of trauma, such as bullying, rejection, or exclusion. These experiences often go beyond mere appearance because they affect our sense of belonging and self-worth, embedding a deep belief that our value is tied to how we look. These obsessive thoughts are not just random; they frequently have roots in these earlier traumas, whether it's feeling ostracized for not fitting in, being judged for our bodies, or absorbing the unspoken message that we are not enough. Understanding that body dysmorphia is frequently tied to these formative experiences can help to contextualize why it feels so deeply ingrained.

The role of stress

Stress is a significant yet often overlooked contributor to body dysmorphia. Prolonged stress, whether from critical environments, work pressure, busyness, or the demands of modern life, keeps the body in a constant state of heightened alertness. Stress changes how our brain functions. The stress response triggers the release of hormones like cortisol and adrenaline which, if prolonged, can impair clear thinking, intensify self-critical thoughts, and drive obsessive behaviours, making it increasingly difficult to escape the cycle of body dysmorphia.

Chronic stress also wears down our ability to cope, blurring the line between past emotional pain and present experiences and trapping the mind in a loop of fear and self-criticism. You begin to carry old insecurities into new situations with stress amplifying them. So, if you're feeling insecure about your body, stress makes those feelings harder to ignore.

The ongoing pressure to meet work or social expectations, combined with personal insecurities, can make things worse. The stress response can fuel a persistent drive to 'fix' perceived flaws as a coping mechanism, controlling the things we can, such as our appearance. This creates a feedback loop where stress feeds body dysmorphia, and body dysmorphia in turn intensifies stress.

Sociocultural pressures

Society and culture play a massive role in shaping body image. The world around us sends constant messages about what an 'ideal' body looks like, and these standards often feel unattainable. Think about the images we're bombarded with on social media – endlessly curated and edited to present perfection. These filtered and flawless representations distort our sense of what's normal and leave us feeling like we're always falling short.

But it's not just about the media. Every culture has its own set of beauty ideals. Depending on your background, you might feel pressure to meet specific standards related to body size, shape, or other physical traits. For example, in some cultures, being thin is glorified, while in others, a more muscular or voluptuous body might be the gold standard. These ever-shifting societal values make it incredibly hard to feel comfortable in your own skin if you don't fit the mould.

The pressure to conform isn't just historical; it's deeply personal and embedded in our daily lives. Whether it's through fashion trends, body-positive movements, or even the ways in which clothing is sized, society's subtle messages shape how we perceive our bodies. One example is vanity sizing, where clothing brands adjust sizes to flatter consumers by labelling larger clothes with smaller size numbers. For instance, what was considered a size 12 several decades ago might now be labelled as a size 8. This distorts our perception of what a 'normal' body size is, reinforcing unrealistic expectations and creating confusion about our bodies, especially when we compare ourselves to outdated standards.

These genetic, environmental, and sociocultural influences intertwine, making body dysmorphia as unique and complex as the individuals who experience it (see Figure 2.2).

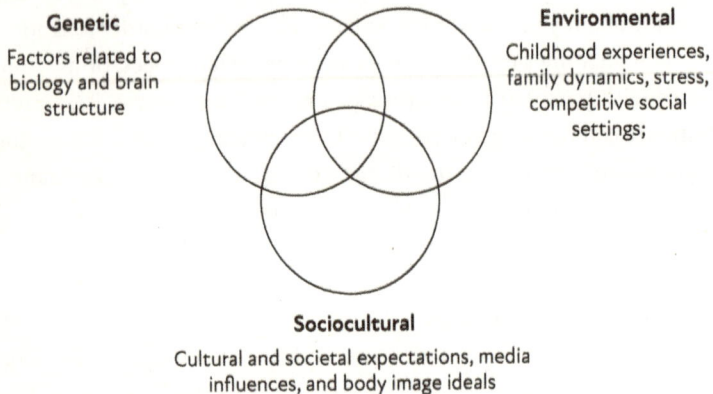

Genetic
Factors related to biology and brain structure

Environmental
Childhood experiences, family dynamics, stress, competitive social settings;

Sociocultural
Cultural and societal expectations, media influences, and body image ideals

Figure 2.2. *Factors contributing to body dysmorphia*

Body dysmorphia in the gay community

Body dysmorphia touches everyone, regardless of gender or sexual orientation. But for gay men, the challenges around body image can be even more intense, magnifying the impact of body dysmorphia. A study found that over 49 per cent of gay and bisexual participants experienced body dysmorphia, significantly higher than their heterosexual counterparts (Schmidt *et al.* 2022). This disparity can be attributed to unique pressures, including fear of rejection, the need to conceal one's sexual orientation, internalized homophobia, stigma, discrimination, and threats of violence.

For gay individuals, these pressures are often compounded by a culture that can be hyper-focused on aesthetics and appearance. The constant exposure to 'ideal' bodies through the media and the community not only affects self-esteem but can also trigger or intensify body dysmorphic tendencies. This combination of societal expectations and internal community pressures creates a unique environment where body image concerns are heightened. For gay men, fitting into mainstream ideals often feels impossible, and within the community, there can be an added layer of scrutiny that makes acceptance even harder to achieve.

The hyper-vigilance that gay men often develop as a protective mechanism in a heteronormative environment can lead to constant self-evaluation of behaviours and body image, especially when exposed to minority stressors. In these circumstances, our bodies become instruments of judgement, making us feel vulnerable, particularly when we do not feel we measure up to these ideals. Additionally, many of us face heightened societal and internal community pressures to achieve a certain physique.

Internalizing masculine ideals

From an early age, society bombards us with expectations of what it means to be a 'real man' – playing with toy guns, avoiding anything deemed feminine, and dressing in blue. Media portrayals of masculinity often showcase action movie heroes, athletes, or wrestlers – lean and muscular men – as the epitome of male attractiveness and success. For gay men, the pressure to live up to these ideals can feel even more intense. It's not just about being fit; it's about proving that we belong.

These masculine ideals are internalized from a young age, reinforcing the pressure to conform to a specific body type. This can lead to an obsession with achieving a physique similar to what we see in the media, even if it's unrealistic. Within the gay community, the emphasis on conforming to a particular body ideal can be intensified because physical appearance often plays a major role in social acceptance and romantic success. Constant comparison to unattainable standards fuels negative self-perception, contributing to body dysmorphia. This struggle is made worse by societal and community pressures, further damaging mental health.

The role of rejection

Rejection – whether from society or even within the gay community – can be a significant factor in how body dysmorphia develops. For many of us, early experiences of exclusion or being told we don't belong leave deep emotional scars. These early encounters with rejection can instil a sense of not being good enough, which often translates into an intense preoccupation with physical appearance, both as a way to gain acceptance and as a numbing behaviour to escape emotional pain.

In the gay community, rejection often manifests in the form of not meeting certain physical ideals. The emphasis on physical attractiveness and the idealization of a particular body type can create an environment where some can feel constantly judged. This external pressure to meet an ideal appearance can lead people to seek validation through their looks, driving an obsession with perceived physical flaws. The need for approval and acceptance within the community drives many to chase physical ideals, often believing that their worth is tied to appearance. While this may provide a temporary boost in self-esteem, it ultimately reinforces the underlying issues of body dysmorphia.

Conversely, within the bear community, there may be social pressure to maintain a larger physique, which can result in feeling compelled to eat more in order to fit in and be accepted. This highlights how body image pressures manifest in different ways across gay subcultures, each with its own set of challenges and expectations.

Research shows that adverse childhood events might be a risk factor for body dysmorphia (Oshana *et al.* 2020). Personal stories from those who have faced bullying or hurtful comments reveal how early rejection can create a cycle of self-criticism and body dissatisfaction. This can lead to obsessive scrutiny of their appearance, possibly as a defence mechanism by the ego to protect itself from future pain and rejection. The endless pursuit of the perfect body is often fuelled by the hope that improving one's appearance will prevent further rejection and bring long-sought acceptance and validation.

The impact of rejection is not just immediate but can have long-term psychological effects, resulting in low self-esteem and body dysmorphia. In response, some may engage in harmful behaviours, believing that achieving a certain look will improve their social standing and self-worth.

Social media

When we scroll through social media, it's easy to forget that what we're seeing isn't real. It's a highlight reel of filtered, edited lives, all designed to trigger a dopamine hit and make us feel like we're missing out. This constant stream of seemingly perfect images can leave us feeling inadequate, exhausted, and suffering from low self-esteem. While social media is now deeply embedded in our lives, offering connection and various benefits, it also presents significant risks for body image and mental health, especially for gay individuals. Platforms like Instagram and Snapchat have been strongly linked to increased body dissatisfaction, eating disorder symptoms, and thoughts about using anabolic steroids (Griffiths *et al.* 2018). Social media exacerbates body image issues by promoting self-objectification and social comparison, with gay and bisexual men particularly susceptible to these pressures due to their higher risk of body image disorders (Filice *et al.* 2020). These findings highlight the double-edged nature of social media, where the pursuit of an idealized self often leads to negative mental health outcomes, reinforcing the importance of mindful and moderated use.

For many gay men, 'thirst traps' – those perfectly staged, attention-grabbing selfies – become the standard we compare ourselves to. We measure our worth against airbrushed, impossible-to-reach images, and it's no surprise that we fall short. The gap between these curated online personas and our real lives can quickly fuel feelings of inadequacy and dissatisfaction with our bodies. To combat the negative effects of social media, it helps to curate your feed to include more diverse body types and take regular digital detoxes to step away from unrealistic standards. This is discussed in detail in Chapter 9.

Shame and trauma

Shame and trauma often play huge roles in how body dysmorphia develops. Early experiences of rejection or ridicule can leave emotional wounds that shape how we see ourselves well into adulthood. These early seeds of rejection are often expressed in unconscious ways, manifesting as negative thoughts, body dysmorphia, anxiety, depression, and obsessive-compulsive behaviours, which are further compounded by internal community pressures.

Research highlights that muscle dysphoria, a subtype of BDD that is a preoccupation with the idea that one's body isn't lean and muscular enough, is correlated with childhood bullying and victimization (Wolke and Sapouna 2008). For many gay men, societal rejection and internalized homophobia intensify these feelings, leading to chronic self-criticism and low self-worth. We'll explore this in more depth in Chapter 4.

Shame, unlike guilt, is entrenched in the perception of oneself as inherently flawed or inadequate. Gay individuals, who may face societal rejection and internalized homophobia, often experience intense shame that can lead to long-term psychological distress. As we grow older, the trauma and shame experienced in our youth can become internalized, manifesting in persistent mental health challenges. Body dysmorphia becomes a way to manage feelings of inadequacy and rejection, with the drive for the 'perfect' body acting as a shield from further rejection or criticism. In an effort to guard against feelings of inadequacy, some may fall into damaging habits, such as strict dieting, obsessive exercise, or dependence on performance-enhancing drugs, all of which take a serious toll on both mental and physical well-being.

Understanding and addressing the influence of shame is crucial for improving mental health and supporting recovery from body dysmorphia among gay individuals. Recognizing the roots of these feelings can help us become more self-aware, breaking free from harmful learnt behaviours formed in childhood. Practising self-compassion, challenging internalized negative beliefs, and building a more supportive community are instruments in healing from body dysmorphia and its comorbidities. This is what we will be discussing in later chapters of this book.

'No fats, no fems' - stigma in the community

Hookup apps are environments where users frequently encounter discriminatory messages, including those that are violent, sexist, ageist, racist, ableist, anti-HIV, and anti-trans. The phrase 'No fats, no fems', commonly found on dating profiles, epitomizes the stigma within the gay community against those who do not fit certain physical ideals. This rejection of overweight and effeminate individuals creates a narrow standard of beauty, leaving many feeling invisible and unworthy if they don't conform. Such messages perpetuate a belief that only a specific type of body is desirable, further deepening the struggles with body dysmorphia.

Additionally, exclusionary phrases like 'clean only' or preferences that specify or exclude certain ethnicities reflect a troubling intersection of preferences that can marginalize people based on their ethnicity, body type, or expression of masculinity. This creates a compounding experience of discrimination for those affected, particularly gay men of colour.

The pressure to look better than their best

Gay men face unique pressures to not only meet but exceed physical expectations, driving them to pursue an often unattainable level of perfection. The desire to look 'better than their best' is often linked to seeking validation and acceptance within the community, where physical appearance plays a significant role in social status and desirability. This is especially visible during high-profile events such as Pride or gay destination vacations, where the pressure to conform to idealized standards becomes amplified.

This societal pressure is not just about looking good but about striving for physical perfection, which can lead to extreme and harmful behaviours, such as overexercising or engaging in dangerous dieting practices. For example, some might be incredibly self-critical for missing a gym session or feel pressured to train excessively to compensate. This pursuit of physical ideals can result in symptoms of burnout and increased stress. Additionally, the pressure to achieve these body ideals may push some towards using anabolic steroids or other performance-enhancing substances to meet community expectations, further intensifying the psychological and physical toll.

Pornography and its influence on body image

The portrayal of the 'perfect body' in pornography often showcases a narrow standard of desirability that many men feel pressured to emulate. This focus on hyper-muscular physiques and enhanced features creates unrealistic expectations, making individuals feel inadequate about their own bodies if they don't match up to these ideals. This doesn't just contribute to body dysmorphia but also fuels genital dysmorphia, with pornography frequently featuring men with larger-than-average genitalia. Genital dysmorphia occurs when there is an obsessive focus on the size and appearance of one's genitals, leading to significant distress. Constant comparisons with the men seen in porn can cause men to develop deeply unrealistic expectations about their bodies, potentially leading them to avoid sexual activity altogether or suffer from performance anxiety. This can have a far-reaching impact on mental health, further complicating the struggles already associated with body dysmorphia.

Acknowledging the unique challenges

The challenges gay men face in relation to body dysmorphia are deeply rooted in societal, cultural, and community-specific pressures. Awareness and support are vital steps in addressing these issues. The gay community must work towards an inclusive and accepting environment that celebrates and respects all body types. Acknowledging the intersection of rejection, past trauma, media influence, and internalized shame, we can begin to dismantle harmful standards that contribute to body dysmorphia and promote healthier, more positive body image for everyone.

Creating a truly inclusive environment means challenging the narrow beauty standards that dominate not only mainstream culture but also the internal perceptions within the gay community. Every member of the community needs to actively participate in fostering acceptance and diversity. By doing this, we can create a space where each individual feels valued and accepted for who they are, irrespective of their physical appearance. When we work together in this way, we create a more positive, supportive, and healing environment that empowers everyone.

The psychological toll of body dysmorphia

Suffering from body dysmorphia is exhausting, particularly for those unaware of their condition or afraid to seek help. The emotional and mental toll of the condition often leads to a range of psychological effects, including obsessive behaviours, anxiety, depression, and social isolation. Furthermore, many develop unhealthy coping mechanisms like disordered eating, including anorexia, bulimia, or binge eating, and may also turn to substance use as an escape.

Obsessive behaviours

Some people with body dysmorphia may exhibit obsessive behaviours focused on their appearance. This can involve excessive grooming, repeated mirror checking, or a compulsive fixation on hiding perceived flaws. Even though these so-called imperfections are often unnoticed by others, the individual spends significant time attempting to 'correct' or hide them.

Body-focused repetitive behaviours, such as skin picking (dermatillomania), hair pulling (trichotillomania), and, in some cases, nail biting (onychophagia) may also develop. These behaviours can become compulsive and difficult to control, often reinforcing the cycle of anxiety and dissatisfaction with one's appearance.

Perfectionism is another manifestation, where individuals are relentlessly self-critical, constantly punishing themselves for any perceived mistake.

Anxiety and depression

Living under constant self-scrutiny and the burden of comparisons can lead to chronic anxiety and depression. For gay people, these feelings are often compounded by societal and community-specific stigma, deepening the cycle of anxiety and despair. This results in a persistent low mood and an overwhelming sense of inadequacy that further fuels body dysmorphia.

Social isolation

Body dysmorphia often results in self-imposed isolation, with individuals withdrawing from social situations due to fear of judgement or rejection. This retreat from social life only worsens the feeling of loneliness and amplifies depression, further deepening the struggle.

Substance use

Some individuals may turn to recreational drugs to cope with the psychological burden of body dysmorphia. However, this can create additional problems. The 'comedown' from substances often leads to intensified feelings of anxiety and depression resulting from chemical imbalances in the brain. Additionally, the potential for addiction to these substances complicates recovery, contributing to the decline in both mental and physical health.

Eating disorders

Unhealthy eating patterns are often closely linked with body dysmorphia, leading to eating disorders such as anorexia, bulimia, or binge eating. While some behaviours arise from the desire to control or change body shape, binge eating may occur as a response to the pressure and emotional distress caused by distorted self-perception and societal expectations to conform to unattainable standards.

Misconceptions

When people confuse body dysmorphia with vanity, they're missing the point entirely. It's not just about wanting to look good – it's a far deeper, more complex issue anchored in psychological distress. Unfortunately, several misconceptions about body dysmorphia, particularly within the gay community, continue to obscure the truth and make it even harder for those affected to get the support they need. Breaking down these misunderstandings is fundamental to a better understanding and building a supportive environment. For example:

- Body dysmorphia is only about weight: One of the biggest myths is that body dysmorphia is just about weight. In reality, body dysmorphia can be about various aspects of physical appearance, including muscle size, body hair, skin texture, and facial features – whatever the individual feels is 'wrong'.
- All gay men are obsessed with their appearance: While societal

pressures and community standards can drive body image issues, not all gay men experience body dysmorphia or place the same emphasis on physical appearance. This stereotype oversimplifies the diversity of experiences and attitudes within the gay community.

- Gay men are vain: The idea that gay men are inherently more focused on their appearance ignores the bigger issue. The pressure to conform to specific physical ideals often stems from deeper struggles with self-worth and acceptance.
- Body dysmorphia in gay men is the same as in heterosexual men: Although body dysmorphia affects people of all sexual orientations, it may be uniquely complicated for gay individuals, given additional stressors like internalized homophobia, discrimination, and aesthetic ideals prevalent in the community. These factors can exacerbate the condition and differentiate it from body dysmorphia in heterosexual men.
- Only young gay men experience body dysmorphia: Body dysmorphia is often associated with youth, but it can affect individuals of any age. Older people may face additional pressures related to ageing and maintaining a youthful appearance, further complicating their relationship with their bodies.
- Body dysmorphia is easily overcome: The idea that body dysmorphia can be 'fixed' through positive thinking underestimates the severity of the condition. It's a serious mental health issue that often requires professional treatment to manage effectively.
- It's just about looking good: At its core, body dysmorphia is not just about appearance but about deeper psychological needs for validation and acceptance. The body becomes a battleground for managing self-esteem, societal pressures, and deeper insecurities.

Different ways people express body dysmorphia

Not everyone experiences or expresses body dysmorphia in the same way. Some people may vocalize their struggles frequently, openly referring to their dissatisfaction with their body and seeking reassurance from others. They might constantly bring up their perceived flaws in conversations, using humour or self-deprecation as a way to express their inner turmoil. This kind of external expression can be a way to manage their feelings of insecurity by receiving validation or sympathy from those around them.

However, for many others, body dysmorphia is a silent battle. Like many mental health conditions, the thoughts and feelings associated with body dysmorphia are kept internal, hidden behind a mask of normalcy. These individuals may appear outwardly composed but are consumed with obsessive thoughts about their appearance. The silence is often driven by fear – fear of being judged, misunderstood, or dismissed as vain. They may also be ashamed of their preoccupation with their appearance, further reinforcing their silence. In some cases, people may not even realize that their constant self-criticism is abnormal, as it feels 'normal' to habitually critique their body. This silent suffering can go unnoticed by friends, family, and even healthcare professionals, making it difficult for individuals to get the help they need. Recognizing that body dysmorphia can be expressed both vocally and quietly is essential for creating understanding and more supportive environments.

Intersectionality

Intersectionality refers to how various aspects of a person's identity – such as ethnicity, gender, sexuality, disability, and health status – combine to create distinct experiences and, in some cases, additional layers of oppression. These overlapping factors can result in particularly unique challenges when it comes to body dysmorphia. For individuals who belong to multiple marginalized groups, the pressures from societal, cultural, and community expectations often intensify the distress associated with body image, creating a more complex and multifaceted experience of the condition.

HIV

HIV can intensify symptoms of body dysmorphia due to the physical and psychological challenges associated with HIV. Those living with HIV might experience significant changes in their bodies due to the virus itself or its treatment, such as weight loss, lipodystrophy (abnormal distribution of body fat), and other visible symptoms. These changes can increase the distress and preoccupation seen in BDD.

Furthermore, the stigma and social discrimination associated with HIV can contribute to or worsen mental health conditions, including body dysmorphia. This can create a vicious cycle where the physical symptoms of HIV and the psychological impact of body dysmorphia amplify each other, leading to greater overall distress.

Neurodiversity

Neurodiversity encompasses a range of neurological differences or neurotypes, including attention deficit hyperactivity disorder (ADHD), autism, dyslexia, dyspraxia, and Tourette syndrome, which can intersect with body dysmorphia in unique and complex ways. Research shows that people with ADHD are more at risk of disordered eating and eating disorders (Levin and Rawana 2016). The struggle with impulsivity and hyper-focus can lead to heightened symptoms of body dysmorphia, such as excessive grooming and mirror checking. This hyper-focus can exacerbate obsessive thoughts about perceived flaws, making it difficult to shift attention away from negative body image. Additionally, emotional dysregulation, common in ADHD, can amplify the distress associated with body dysmorphia, leading to heightened anxiety and depression.

People with autism may experience body dysmorphia differently due to unique sensory sensitivities and heightened focus on detail. This can result in intense preoccupation with specific aspects of their appearance. Social communication challenges often experienced by autistic individuals can lead to social isolation, further exacerbating feelings of loneliness and depression commonly associated with body dysmorphia. The rigidity in thinking and difficulty with change that many autistic individuals experience can make it harder for them to adapt to body changes or accept imperfections.

Both ADHD and autism can involve difficulties with executive functioning, impacting the ability to maintain consistent self-care routines and seek treatment for body dysmorphia. Poor executive functioning can also lead to impulsive behaviours, such as binge eating or excessive exercising, as coping mechanisms. Additionally, the allure of controlled nutrition, such as calorie counting or restricting food groups, can create hyper-focus in someone with ADHD or be particularly appealing to an autistic person. The social and interpersonal challenges faced by those with ADHD and autism, such as maintaining relationships and effective communication, can compound the isolation felt by those with body dysmorphia.

When considering treatment approaches that address both neuro-diversity and body dysmorphia, sensitivity is essential and an approach that takes into account both conditions is crucial. This might include medication for managing ADHD symptoms, cognitive-behavioural therapy (CBT) for body dysmorphia, and strategies to improve executive functioning. It is important to recognize that treatment aims to address specific challenges and enhance quality of life rather than trying to 'fix' the neurotype itself. Understanding the intersection of neurodiversity and body dysmorphia is essential for providing effective support and promoting a more inclusive and supportive environment where neurodiverse individuals are accepted and celebrated.

Culture and ethnicity

A person's ethnic background can deeply influence their experience with body dysmorphia. In many societies, certain beauty standards are more prominently represented, leaving people from diverse ethnic and cultural backgrounds feeling under-represented or pressured to fit these ideals. This lack of representation can make it difficult for those who don't see themselves reflected in the dominant beauty narrative, adding extra challenges for those already struggling with body dysmorphia.

For gay men of colour, this can be especially challenging. They may face a complex mix of expectations – both from mainstream culture and from within their own communities – which can intensify feelings of not measuring up. This can lead to a heightened sense of body dissatisfaction as they navigate a unique set of pressures related to their appearance and identity.

Recovery

Recovery from body dysmorphia is a complex and personal journey that extends beyond simply addressing physical symptoms. It involves a deep, holistic process of self-acceptance, confronting and dealing with underlying traumas, and making meaningful changes to both mindset and daily habits. Recovery is about transforming how you perceive and relate to your body, developing healthier coping mechanisms, and building a supportive environment where you feel you belong.

My recovery journey hasn't been straightforward. I can still easily look in the mirror and begin the self-critical narrative, be harder on myself than ever, and even have fantasies about using anabolic steroids again. Some days are better than others. When I began my recovery, I had to be completely honest with myself. It was so easy for me to focus on worrying about others as a distraction technique to avoid doing the work myself. I wasn't even aware I was doing this – and being a nutritionist, this came as second nature to me. My experiences with psychedelics served as a tool to hold up a compassionate mirror, helping me understand who I really am and what work needs to be done to heal from all the trauma I have experienced in life. This also involved accepting myself wholly, embracing my shadow, and understanding the parts of myself that I had previously neglected or hidden away. It means integrating all aspects of my identity and experiences, both positive and negative, into a cohesive and accepting self-view.

The road ahead can be challenging and may include setbacks and days when you are triggered, feel overwhelmed, and have many moments of doubt. However, it's important to remember that these obstacles are part of the process. Recovery is not linear, and it's okay to experience ups and downs along the way.

This book will be your companion on the road ahead, with each chapter dedicated to a different pillar of body dysmorphia recovery, which includes:

- Nutrition: Examining the role of diet in mental health and body image. Understanding the biochemical links between food, mood, and self-perception and developing a balanced and supportive approach to eating to nourish the body.
- Trauma: Addressing and healing from past traumas that contribute to body dysmorphia. Exploring therapeutic approaches and self-help strategies to deal with emotional pain and its impact on body image.
- Mindset: Shifting your mental framework to create self-compassion, resilience, and a positive body image. This involves

challenging destructive self-criticism and cultivating nurturing thought patterns.

- Movement: Discovering physical activities that you enjoy and that support your body positively, without the pressure of achieving a perfect physique. Emphasizing the joy of movement and the benefits of exercise as a form of self-care.
- Stillness: Incorporating practices like meditation and mindfulness to create inner peace and reduce stress. Learning to appreciate the value of stillness and solitude in healing and self-acceptance.
- Building a supportive environment: Creating a network of supportive relationships and safe spaces that encourage and sustain your recovery journey. This includes friends, family, and professionals who understand and support your healing process.

Each of these pillars will be explored in depth, providing you with practical strategies and insights to navigate your path to recovery and build a healthier relationship with your body and self. My advice is to read through this book first and then return to the section you wish to begin with. The important thing is not to feel overloaded with information; change should be gradual and manageable. Perhaps start by implementing one or two changes per week. This could be as simple as incorporating a new mindful movement practice or beginning a daily meditation routine. Allow yourself time to settle into these changes before adding more. This approach ensures that each new habit becomes a sustainable part of your life rather than a fleeting attempt at improvement. Recovery is a marathon, not a sprint, and it's essential to pace yourself and celebrate small victories along the way.

By taking it slow and steady, you give yourself the best chance at lasting change and a deeper, more resilient recovery. This gradual approach helps to build confidence and ensures that you are not overwhelmed by trying to do too much at once. Remember, it's the cumulative effect of small, consistent changes that leads to significant and lasting transformation.

Exercise: Understanding self-criticism

Part 1: Understanding your self-criticism

Take a moment to reflect on the specific ways in which you are hard on yourself. Write down the common criticisms you have about yourself. These could be related to your appearance, performance, relationships, or any other aspect of your life. Next, think about where these critical thoughts come from. Are they influenced by past experiences, societal expectations, or comparisons with others? Write down any insights about the origins of your self-criticism.

Consider how these critical thoughts affect you. Do they motivate you, or do they hold you back? Write a few sentences about how being hard on yourself impacts on your emotional well-being, relationships, and overall quality of life.

Part 2: Imagining a kinder approach

Imagine what your life would be like if you were less hard on yourself. How would your daily experiences change if you approached yourself with kindness and understanding instead of criticism? Write down what comes to mind in this imagined scenario, particularly paying attention to any resistance that comes to mind.

List the potential benefits of being kinder to yourself. Consider aspects such as improved mental health, stronger relationships, increased motivation, and a greater sense of inner peace. Think about small, actionable steps you can take to be less critical and more compassionate towards yourself. Write down at least three specific actions you can implement in your daily life to cultivate self-compassion.

The aim of this exercise is to begin the process of self-enquiry and go beyond the surface of your self-critical tendencies. When you imagine a kinder approach, you can uncover the deeper impacts of self-criticism on your life and explore the potential benefits of self-compassion. This reflection will help you understand how treating yourself with more kindness can lead to improved mental health, stronger relationships, and a greater sense of inner peace.

CHAPTER 3

The Role of Nutrition in Body Dysmorphia

NUTRITION IS A SENSITIVE AREA IN REGARD TO BODY DYSMOR-PHIA. Many of us are familiar with the principles of dieting, often using restriction or control to achieve specific goals or as a form of self-punishment. In body dysmorphia, the relationship with food can become even more complex, as nutritional choices may be tied to deeper issues around self-worth and body image. Navigating nutrition and lifestyle changes can be particularly challenging in this context. It is essential to strike a balance between providing proper nourishment and avoiding an overly controlled or restrictive approach, which could potentially worsen symptoms of body dysmorphia. It's not just about what we eat but why we eat. Food can become a comfort, a punishment, or a form of control when our emotional needs aren't being met. Recognizing these patterns is key to building a healthier, more balanced relationship with nutrition.

With this in mind, this chapter not only provides instructional advice on how to balance your nutrition but also explores the intricate connection between nutrition and mental health, especially within the context of body dysmorphia. My goal is to supply an understanding of the pivotal role that diet plays in maintaining and improving well-being. By equipping yourself with the right tools, my hope is that you can take proactive steps towards better psychological health, which may manifest in a more balanced mind and greater self-esteem.

Getting started

I appreciate that this chapter is quite technical, but it's important to give you all the variables at play in regard to body dysmorphia. Understanding these factors will empower you to make informed decisions about your diet and overall health. As you read through this chapter, make note of what is relevant to you. There is a 'Creating a personalized nutrition plan' section to help you put things together.

Remember that this chapter is designed to provide you with information without overwhelming you. If you find yourself unsure where to begin or feeling the need to do everything at once, my advice is to take a step back. Start with two or three simple changes that you can make to your schedule, making sure they are sustainable. For instance, you might start by adding more protein, incorporating more vegetables into your meals, and ensuring you stay hydrated throughout the day.

Adopt an 'I'll get there' approach, especially if you tend to be hard on yourself for not being perfect. The journey ahead will have its ups and downs, and there will be times when your diet may not go as planned. With a compassionate approach to nutrition, you will find it easier to go with the flow, are more likely to nourish yourself effectively, and healthy eating will eventually become second nature.

Remember, it's okay to seek support from friends, support groups, a professional, or a therapist, if needed. Creating a support system can provide encouragement and companionship, making the process less daunting and more achievable.

Ultimately, the goal is to develop a personalized nutrition plan that supports your mental and physical health, helping you create a more loving and sustainable relationship with your body that lasts.

Shifting away from diets and restrictions

My aim in writing this chapter is to embed within your subconscious a shift away from diets and restrictions to a more nourishing mindset, where eating healthily becomes habitual, enjoyable, and something you naturally gravitate towards. This approach helps to avoid things like binge eating while allowing flexibility and not demonizing any particular food or food groups. This may seem quite challenging to read at first, but my hope is that it becomes easier as you work through other chapters in this book. Addressing underlying emotional health, trauma, and mindset allows you to take a broader perspective on diet and nutrition. This understanding helps you to recognize what will work for you and identify potential triggers. Additionally, it enables you to sit with your thoughts and feelings rather than reaching for convenience food or alcohol if you are feeling stressed, preoccupied, or overwhelmed. We will take a deep dive into these topics in Chapters 4 and 5.

Blood sugar balance

Blood sugar, or blood glucose, is the main sugar found in the blood and comes from the food we eat. It's the body's primary source of energy and is crucial for proper bodily functions. When you eat carbohydrates, they are broken down into glucose, which then enters the bloodstream. The hormone insulin, produced by the pancreas, helps cells absorb this glucose to be used for energy. When blood sugar levels drop, the hormone glucagon signals the liver to release stored glucose to maintain balance. While carbohydrates are the most direct source of glucose, proteins and fats can also be converted into glucose through metabolic processes, although this occurs more slowly.

Maintaining stable blood sugar levels is vital for overall health (see Figure 3.1). Rapid fluctuations can lead to various symptoms, such as fatigue, mood swings, and food cravings, and over time, can contribute to more serious health issues like insulin resistance, metabolic syndrome, and type 2 diabetes.

The importance of blood sugar balance in body dysmorphia

For individuals with body dysmorphia, stable blood sugar levels are particularly important. Fluctuating blood sugar can exacerbate mood swings, anxiety, and stress, which can intensify body image issues. Additionally, erratic eating patterns, such as skipping meals or consuming high-sugar foods, can lead to these fluctuations, further complicating mental health and body image perceptions.

Balancing blood sugar helps to create a more stable emotional state and reduces the physiological stress that can exacerbate body dysmorphia. This balance can aid in managing cravings and avoiding the binge–restrict cycle often associated with body image issues.

Maintaining stable blood sugar levels also contributes to healthier skin. Fluctuating blood sugar can lead to increased inflammation and insulin spikes, which may contribute to skin issues like acne. Studies have shown that high-glycaemic diets can exacerbate acne by increasing insulin levels and androgen activity, leading to greater sebum production and inflammation (Smith *et al.* 2007). When you keep your blood sugar balanced, you support overall skin health and help maintain a clearer complexion. Clear and healthy skin can significantly impact self-esteem and body image, reducing one area of potential stress and concern.

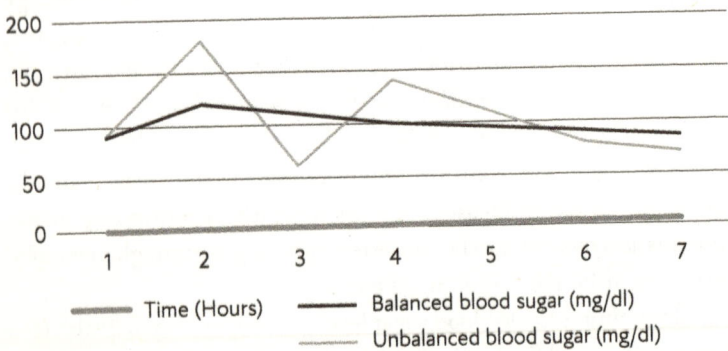

Figure 3.1. *Comparison of balanced vs. unbalanced blood sugar levels over time*

Blood sugar balance vs. dieting

Unlike traditional dieting, which often involves restrictive practices and calorie counting, focusing on blood sugar balance promotes a sustainable and holistic approach to nutrition, supporting long-term well-being. Traditional diets can lead to short-term weight loss but are often hard to maintain and can result in a cycle of restriction and overeating. This can be particularly harmful for those with body dysmorphia, as the failure to adhere to strict diets can cause feelings of inadequacy and body dissatisfaction.

In contrast, balancing blood sugar emphasizes regular, balanced meals that include a variety of nutrients. This approach avoids the extreme highs and lows in energy levels that can trigger cravings and mood swings. It focuses on:

- Stability: Maintaining steady blood sugar levels throughout the day helps in achieving a more balanced mood and energy state.
- Nourishment: Ensuring the body gets a consistent supply of nutrients to support overall health and well-being.
- Natural weight maintenance: Balancing blood sugar naturally supports weight maintenance by reducing insulin spikes and crashes, which helps to control appetite and prevent overeating. Consistent energy levels prevent cravings for high-sugar and high-fat foods, leading to healthier food choices. Additionally, this balance encourages the body to burn stored fat for energy rather than storing excess calories as fat, promoting gradual and sustainable weight loss.
- Bulking: It's also possible to support muscle gain through blood sugar balance. Through maintaining steady blood sugar levels and avoiding spikes and crashes, individuals can ensure they have the energy needed for intense workouts and proper muscle recovery. Consuming balanced meals with adequate protein, healthy fats, and complex carbohydrates helps build muscle mass while preventing fat accumulation.
- Sustainability: A balanced approach to eating that can be maintained long term without feelings of deprivation or the risk of binge eating.

How to balance blood sugar

Balancing blood sugar involves both dietary and lifestyle adjustments. Some key strategies include the following:

- Add protein to each meal and snack: Protein slows down the digestion of carbohydrates and the release of sugar into the blood. Good sources include lean meats, fish, eggs, dairy, legumes, tofu, tempeh, nuts, and seeds.
- Opt for complex carbohydrates: Wholemeal bread, brown rice, quinoa, and oats are examples of complex carbohydrates. These

are digested more slowly than refined carbohydrates, helping to maintain stable blood sugar levels.

- Include healthy fats: The presence of fat in a meal can help moderate blood sugar spikes. Good sources of fats include avocados, nuts, seeds, olive oil, and oily fish.
- Reduce refined sugars: Avoid foods and drinks high in refined sugars, which cause rapid spikes and drops in blood sugar. Instead, focus on foods with natural sugars, such as fruit, and those that release sugar slowly into the bloodstream. When shopping, it's helpful to check food labels to spot hidden sugars, particularly in processed foods.
- Hydrate: Drinking plenty of water throughout the day can support stable blood sugar levels. Aim for 2–3 litres of fluid per day, and consider herbal teas and water flavoured with lemon or cucumber if plain water is unappealing.
- Limit caffeine and alcohol: Both can affect blood sugar levels in some individuals. Moderation is important, so water, decaffeinated beverages, de-alcoholized drinks, or herbal teas may be beneficial substitutes.
- Manage stress: Stress increases the hormone cortisol, which can disrupt blood sugar balance. Practices like mindfulness, meditation, and regular physical activity can help manage stress levels.
- Regular physical activity: Exercise improves insulin sensitivity and helps maintain stable blood sugar levels. Aim for a mix of aerobic exercise, strength training, and flexibility exercises.
- Adequate sleep: Aim for 7–9 hours of quality sleep per night to maintain a healthy balance of blood sugar levels. Poor sleep can negatively impact blood sugar and overall health.
- Avoid skipping meals: This can lead to blood sugar drops and subsequent overeating. Regular, balanced meals help maintain stable blood sugar levels.

Sample blood sugar balancing day
Breakfast
Overnight oats: Combine rolled oats, chia seeds, and unsweetened almond milk in a jar. Let it sit overnight in the fridge. In the morning, top with Greek yoghurt, nuts, fresh berries and a drizzle of honey (optional).

Mid-morning snack
Apple slices with almond butter: Slice the apple and serve with almond butter for dipping.

Lunch
Quinoa salad with grilled chicken: Mix cooked quinoa with mixed greens, cherry tomatoes, cucumber, and avocado. Top with sliced grilled chicken breast. Drizzle with olive oil and lemon juice, and season with salt and pepper.

Afternoon snack
Hummus with veggie sticks: Serve hummus with sliced cucumber, bell peppers, and carrots for a crunchy, savoury option.

Dinner
Salmon with steamed vegetables and brown rice: Marinate the salmon fillet with olive oil, lemon juice, and minced garlic. Bake at 190°C (375°F) for about 20 minutes or until cooked through. Serve with steamed vegetables and a side of brown rice.

Evening snack
Mixed berries and cottage cheese: Mix berries with cottage cheese for a satisfying and protein-rich snack.

Understanding macronutrients: carbohydrates, proteins, and fats

Carbohydrates

Carbohydrates are the body's primary source of energy. They are broken down into glucose, which is used by the body's cells for fuel. Carbohydrates can be categorized into simple and complex carbs.

- Simple carbohydrates: Quick to digest and provide immediate energy but can cause rapid spikes in blood sugar. Examples: table sugar, honey, fruit juice, sweets, confectionery.
- Complex carbohydrates: Digested more slowly, providing a steady release of energy and helping to maintain stable blood sugar levels. Examples: whole grains (brown rice, quinoa, oats), vegetables, legumes (lentils, beans).

Proteins

Proteins are made up of smaller building blocks called amino acids. Proteins are essential for building and repairing tissues, making enzymes and hormones, and supporting overall body function. They also play a role in maintaining satiety and supporting blood sugar balance by slowing the digestion of carbohydrates.

- Animal-based proteins: Generally complete proteins providing all essential amino acids. Examples: chicken, fish, eggs, dairy products (milk, cheese, yoghurt).
- Plant-based proteins: Often incomplete proteins but can be combined to provide all essential amino acids. Examples: beans, lentils, tofu, quinoa, nuts, seeds.

Fats

Fats are a concentrated source of energy and are essential for absorbing fat-soluble vitamins (A, D, E, K), protecting organs, and maintaining cell membranes. They also help slow digestion and maintain stable blood sugar levels.

- Healthy fats: Beneficial for heart health and overall well-being. Examples: avocados, nuts, seeds, olive oil, fatty fish (salmon, mackerel).
- Saturated fats: Can be part of a healthy diet when consumed in moderation. Examples: fatty cuts of meat, butter, cheese, coconut oil.
- Unhealthy fats: Should be limited due to their potential negative effects on health, particularly trans fats. Examples: trans fats (partially hydrogenated oils found in many processed foods), excessive saturated fats (found in fatty cuts of meat, butter, cheese).

Sugar, caffeine, and ultra-processed foods

Diets high in sugar, caffeine, and ultra-processed foods can have negative effects on mood and energy levels, particularly for individuals with body dysmorphia. These substances contribute to fluctuations in blood sugar levels, leading to periods of irritability, anxiety, and fatigue. For example, consuming a sugary snack may provide a quick burst of energy, but it is often followed by a sharp drop, leaving one feeling fatigued and irritable. Likewise, while caffeine can temporarily boost alertness, excessive intake can result in jitteriness, disrupted sleep, and increased anxiety. This effect is further compounded if you are adding sugar to your beverages.

In body dysmorphia, these mood swings and energy crashes can heighten feelings of dissatisfaction and stress related to body image. Ultra-processed foods, which often contain high levels of unhealthy fats, sugars, and additives, can further amplify these issues, creating a cycle where the temporary relief provided by these foods is quickly followed by negative physical and emotional repercussions. Over time, this cycle can intensify symptoms of anxiety and depression, making it more difficult to maintain a balanced and positive self-perception.

Ultimately, the mood instability and energy fluctuations caused by these dietary choices can manifest as heightened body dysmorphia symptoms. Some may become more critical of their appearance, experience increased anxiety about their body image, and find it challenging to break free from obsessive thoughts about perceived flaws, especially if these foods lead to weight gain or exacerbate skin conditions such as acne. Limiting the intake of sugar, caffeine, and processed foods can help you achieve more stable energy levels and a balanced mood, which is crucial for managing stress and anxiety associated with body image issues.

The diet trap

Many people with body dysmorphia have a history of dieting or restricting food in a quest for the 'perfect body'. I usually tell my clients that most diets work if you stick to them, which underscores the very essence of the problem – not blaming the individual but recognizing that most diet plans are unsustainable and overly restrictive. Dieting with body dysmorphia is complex because there are significant psychological factors involved. Starting a diet can initially provide a sense of control, confidence, and motivation. However, the inevitable slip-ups can lead to feelings of failure and guilt, resulting in disastrous emotional consequences and further exacerbating body dysmorphia.

Moreover, the rigid structure of many diets can actually make the situation worse. These diets often impose strict rules and limitations that are difficult to maintain over the long term. When individuals are unable to adhere to these demanding guidelines, they may experience heightened stress and anxiety, which can negatively affect their mental health. This stress can also trigger unhealthy eating behaviours, such as binge eating or extreme restriction, leading to physical health issues like nutrient deficiencies or metabolic imbalances. Thus, the inflexible nature of dieting not only fails to address the underlying issues of body dysmorphia but also adds further layers of complexity to the problem, impacting overall well-being.

I was drawn into diet culture at a young age, believing that the stricter the diet, the better I would feel. I gaslighted myself into thinking I was doing wonders for my body, even as I felt drained during restrictive phases, whether fasting or cutting out carbohydrates. I was great at adhering to a diet during the structured weekdays, but when the weekend came, I often fell off the waggon, especially after having a few drinks. Once I crossed my threshold for what I considered over-indulgence, I convinced myself that the diet was ruined, and I'd start again on Monday. This mindset permitted me to binge eat anything and everything because I believed I'd start afresh with restrictions on Monday. This created a constant cycle of shame, obsessively scruti-nizing my body, and being overly critical of myself for breaking the diet – all because I thought I looked fat in the mirror. I put immense pressure on myself to be ready for the next holiday, party, or even to feel slightly more comfortable during sex.

The downside of calorie counting

Calorie counting is a common practice in many diet plans and is often seen as a straightforward way to manage weight. However, this practice can become an unhealthy obsession. Constantly tracking every calorie can lead to an overly restrictive mindset and increase anxiety around food choices. It reduces the complex nature of nutrition to mere num-bers, ignoring the importance of food quality and overall health. This fixation on calories can overshadow the body's actual nutritional needs, leading to further imbalances and keeping you in a cycle of restriction and guilt when calorie targets are not met.

Research has shown that dieting can lead to higher levels of cortisol (Tomiyama *et al.* 2010), which not only affects mood but also pro-motes fat storage, counteracting the purpose and goal of dieting. Die-tary restrictions can also overshadow the importance of nutrition and health, possibly leading to nutritional deficiencies and poorer health outcomes. This can lead to symptoms including lethargy, a weakened immune system, hair loss, or skin changes, further complicating phys-ical and mental health and exacerbating body dysmorphia.

Treat and cheat meals

Incorporating relaxed meals or days into a balanced eating plan can be particularly relevant for individuals with body dysmorphia. I dis-courage use of the terminology 'treat' or 'cheat', as this often implies you're doing something wrong or that certain foods are rewards, which can create a dichotomy of 'good' and 'bad' foods. This polarized thinking can magnify feelings of guilt and shame when consuming such foods and reinforce a negative relationship with food. By reframing these occasions as relaxed meals or days, we avoid demonizing specific foods.

Having a relaxed meal is about finding a healthy balance between enjoying the foods you desire and maintaining overall dietary goals. It's important to approach these meals with a positive frame of mind, viewing them as part of a sustainable lifestyle rather than a deviation from a strict diet. This mindset helps in reducing the psychological stress associated with food restriction and promotes a more inclusive perspective on eating.

When planning a relaxed meal, consider the following:

- Mindful enjoyment: Take the time to savour and enjoy your food. Eating mindfully can enhance your satisfaction and prevent overindulgence.
- Portion control: Enjoy the foods you love in moderation. This allows you to indulge without feeling like you've sabotaged your health goals.
- Balance: Incorporate relaxed meals into your overall balanced diet. Ensure that the rest of your meals are nutrient-dense and health-focused.
- No guilt: Remind yourself that it's okay to enjoy all types of food. While it is very easy to slip into feeling guilty, try to avoid doing so about your choices, as this can lead to a negative cycle of restriction and bingeing.
- Listen to your body: Pay attention to how your body feels before, during, and after the meal. Eating what you desire should make you feel satisfied and happy, not uncomfortable or regretful.
- Check your motivation: Before indulging, ask yourself if you truly want the food or if you're eating out of habit or for emotional reasons. Recognize any thoughts of self-sabotage and address them by focusing on making mindful, intentional choices that support your well-being.

Biological factors affecting body dysmorphia
Hunger hormones

Dieting also has an impact on hunger hormones such as leptin and ghrelin, which regulate appetite and satiety. Leptin signals to the brain to stop eating when you are full, while ghrelin stimulates appetite. Restrictive diets can disrupt the balance of these hormones, making you hungrier and less satisfied even after eating. This hormonal imbalance can lead to overeating and weight gain once the diet is over, keeping alive the cycle of dieting, body dissatisfaction, and psychological stress.

Leptin resistance

A more complex issue arises when someone develops leptin resistance. Leptin resistance is a condition where the body's cells become less responsive to leptin, leading to impaired signalling to the brain about fullness. Despite having high levels of leptin, those with leptin resistance do not feel satiated after eating, which can lead to overeating and weight gain. Chronic dieting and obesity are commonly linked to leptin resistance, which increases feelings of dissatisfaction and further contributes to body dysmorphia.

Several factors may disrupt leptin function and contribute to resistance, including:

- Chronic inflammation: Inflammatory signals can interfere with leptin signalling in the brain.
- High levels of free fatty acids: Excess fatty acids in the bloodstream can increase inflammation and disrupt leptin signalling.
- High-sugar intake: Diets high in sugar, especially fructose, can impair leptin function.
- Poor sleep: Poor sleep can lower leptin levels and increase ghrelin levels, leading to increased hunger.

Ghrelin's impact

Ghrelin increases before meals, signalling the need to eat. After dieting, ghrelin levels can remain elevated, making it harder to feel satisfied and increasing the risk of overeating. This is why many people regain weight after restrictive diets, creating a frustrating cycle of body dissatisfaction and further dieting attempts.

Supporting healthy hunger hormones

Balancing leptin and ghrelin through diet and lifestyle changes is essential for maintaining a healthy appetite and preventing overeating. Here are some foods and strategies to encourage healthy hunger hormones:

- Protein-rich foods: Protein promotes satiety hormones and reduces ghrelin levels, supporting appetite regulation.
- Healthy fats: Omega-3 fatty acids, found in fatty fish (like salmon and sardines), flaxseeds, chia seeds, and walnuts, reduce inflammation and support leptin sensitivity.
- Fibre-rich foods: Foods high in fibre, such as fruit, vegetables, whole grains, and legumes, slow digestion and promote fullness, helping to regulate ghrelin levels.
- Whole foods: Focus on whole, unprocessed foods that provide essential nutrients and support overall health, which can improve leptin sensitivity.
- Anti-inflammatory foods: Foods like berries, leafy greens, and nuts can help reduce inflammation and support healthy leptin function.
- Adequate sleep and physical activity: Prioritizing sleep and regular exercise improves leptin sensitivity and maintains hormonal balance.

Addressing these biological factors helps you to take a more sustainable approach to managing hunger, improving body image, and creating a more positive relationship with food. Most likely, if you are following a blood sugar balancing diet, it will naturally cover many of these aspects, helping to regulate hunger hormones and support overall well-being.

Thyroid function and weight loss

Alongside hunger hormones, thyroid function also plays a critical role in weight management. The thyroid regulates metabolism through hormones like thyroxine (T4) and triiodothyronine (T3), which control how efficiently the body burns calories. Impaired thyroid function, such as in hypothyroidism, can slow metabolism, leading to weight gain or difficulty losing weight. Even mild thyroid dysfunction can make weight management more challenging, contributing to body dissatisfaction and further complicating efforts to maintain a balanced self-image. A simple blood test can assess thyroid function and can be requested through your doctor or a private clinic.

Testosterone

Testosterone plays a vital role in muscle mass, fat distribution, metabolism, mood stability, and libido, all of which impact body image and self-esteem. Low testosterone is often overlooked in discussions about body dysmorphia, but its effects can contribute significantly to body dissatisfaction, fatigue, and difficulty maintaining muscle mass, leading some individuals to engage in extreme dieting or overtraining in an attempt to compensate.

Causes of low testosterone

Testosterone levels naturally decline with age, but several factors can contribute to low levels, including:

- Chronic stress: Elevated cortisol levels can suppress testosterone production.
- Poor sleep: Sleep deprivation is linked to lower testosterone levels and increased hunger hormones.
- Nutritional deficiencies: Low zinc, vitamin D, and magnesium levels can impair testosterone production.
- Excessive dieting or overtraining: Caloric restriction and excessive exercise can disrupt hormonal balance.
- Body composition: Carrying excess body fat, particularly around the abdomen, may contribute to hormonal imbalances, including lower testosterone levels.
- Alcohol and drug use: Frequent or heavy use of alcohol, anabolic steroids, or certain recreational drugs may affect hormone balance and contribute to lower testosterone levels over time.

Signs of low testosterone

- Loss of muscle mass and strength.
- Increased body fat, especially around the abdomen.
- Low energy, mood swings, and reduced motivation.
- Decreased libido and sexual function.

(Bhasin et al. 2018; Hackett et al. 2023)

How to support healthy testosterone levels

- Prioritize sleep: Aim for 7–9 hours per night.
- Ensure enough calories from a nutrient-rich diet: Focus on foods rich in zinc (red meat, shellfish, nuts), magnesium (leafy greens, seeds, whole grains), and vitamin D (sunlight, oily fish, fortified foods). Include healthy fats from eggs, avocados, nuts, and fatty fish to support hormone production.
- Incorporate strength training: Resistance workouts naturally boost testosterone.
- Manage stress: Practise mindfulness, relaxation techniques, and proper recovery.

A blood test can assess your testosterone levels, which can be arranged through a doctor or private clinic. In some cases, testosterone replacement therapy may be an option, but this should always be discussed with a medical professional.

Downfalls of trying to put on weight

On the flip side, some individuals may struggle with the pressure to put on weight and muscle mass. This often involves following high-calorie diets and intensive workout regimes. However, these efforts can also be fraught with challenges and setbacks.

Many people trying to gain weight may find themselves consuming large amounts of food, which can be mentally and physically exhausting. The pressure to eat beyond natural hunger cues can lead to discomfort, digestive issues, and an unhealthy relationship with food. Just like with dieting, trying to gain weight can lead to an overemphasis on certain macronutrients, such as protein and carbohydrates, at the expense of a balanced diet. This can result in nutrient deficiencies, imbalanced blood sugar, and other health issues.

Additionally, there is often significant guilt associated with missing meals or not meeting daily caloric targets. This guilt can lead to stress and anxiety, similar to the feelings experienced by those trying to lose weight. The constant pressure to eat and the fear of not consuming enough calories can make the process of gaining weight just as mentally taxing as restrictive dieting.

The obsession with meal timing and portion sizes can strengthen body dysmorphia. The fear of losing progress or not reaching weight goals can dominate thoughts, leading to a preoccupation with food that disrupts daily life and mental health.

Diet sustainability

Recognizing the unsustainable nature of restrictive diets and the importance of a balanced, flexible approach to eating can support both physical and mental health and a better relationship with food. Finding a sustainable eating pattern that fits your lifestyle and preferences is crucial rather than following restrictive diets that are hard to maintain. A sustainable diet is one that you can stick to long term without feeling deprived or stressed. This involves making gradual changes to your eating habits, focusing on whole, nutrient-dense foods, and allowing yourself the flexibility to enjoy all types of foods in moderation. Emphasizing sustainability can help shift the focus from short-term weight loss to long-term health and well-being. This approach not only supports physical health but also promotes a healthier relationship with food and body image.

Nutrition and mental health

When I released my first book, *Naked Nutrition* (which is now being rewritten as *The Queer Guide to Nutrition and Lifestyle*), the most common retort was, 'Why do LGBTQ+ individuals have different nutrition needs?' Rather than suggesting not to judge a book by its cover, I explained that nutrition encompasses so much more than weight loss and disease prevention. Nutrition plays a vital role in our overall well-being, influencing everything from our energy levels to our mental health. It's not just about calories or nutrients; it's about how food can nourish, heal, and support our body and mind in a holistic way.

What we eat can have a significant effect on our mood, cognitive function, and emotional well-being. The connection between diet and mental health is supported by growing research, highlighting that a balanced, nutrient-rich diet can help to improve mental health outcomes and support overall well-being (Firth *et al.* 2020; Grajek *et al.* 2022).

The relationship between nutrition and mental health is complex, involving numerous factors that influence each other. When you go on a diet and lose weight, you often feel better and more content with your body, which can contribute to improved mental health. Eating well can also help prevent chronic health conditions that might otherwise trigger poor mental health if experienced. Nutrition can act as a form of therapy for mental health conditions, supporting overall mood and well-being. For example, deficiencies in certain nutrients, such as specific fats, vitamins, and minerals, can negatively impact mental health, while a diet rich in lean protein, complex carbohydrates, fruit, and vegetables can protect it.

It is essential to approach mental health from a holistic perspective, recognizing that it encompasses not only emotional and psychological factors but also biological and nutritional ones. Considering the impact of diet and lifestyle on mental well-being allows us to identify key areas where nutritional changes can make a meaningful difference. This comprehensive approach enables us to target the underlying causes of body image concerns rather than just managing the symptoms, offering a more sustainable path to mental and physical health.

Additionally, making thoughtful food choices can contribute to greater mental balance, which in turn supports broader efforts to improve mental health. This is especially important with body dysmorphia, as a balanced diet can help reduce the intense mood swings and emotional fluctuations often tied to body image issues, encouraging a more stable and positive sense of self.

Neurotransmitters

One of the key ways nutrition influences mental health is through the production of neurotransmitters and the balance of hormones. The foods we consume have a direct impact on the production of neurotransmitters – chemicals that transmit signals in the brain. They play a critical role in regulating mood, sleep, and cognitive function. Examples of neurotransmitters include serotonin, dopamine, and norepinephrine. Hormones, which are produced by various glands in the body, also play a significant role in regulating mood and stress levels.

The production of these neurotransmitters and hormones depends heavily on the nutrients we obtain from our diet. For instance, certain amino acids, vitamins, and minerals act as building blocks for neurotransmitters. Without adequate nutrition, the body cannot produce these essential chemicals effectively, leading to imbalances that can affect mental health.

Specific foods that support neurotransmitter health

- Tryptophan-rich foods: Tryptophan is an essential amino acid that the body uses to produce serotonin, often referred to as the 'feel-good' neurotransmitter due to its role in promoting feelings of well-being and happiness. Foods high in tryptophan include turkey, eggs, cheese, nuts, and seeds.
- Tyrosine-rich foods: Tyrosine is another amino acid important for the production of dopamine, a neurotransmitter associated with pleasure and reward. Foods rich in tyrosine include chicken, fish, dairy products, avocados, and bananas.
- Omega-3 fatty acids: These are key for brain health and can support the production of neurotransmitters. As shared earlier in the chapter, they can be found in fatty fish (salmon, mackerel, sardines), flaxseeds, chia seeds, and walnuts.
- B vitamins: These vitamins, particularly B6, B12, and folate,

are essential for neurotransmitter synthesis and overall brain health. Leafy greens, beans, and whole grains are excellent sources of B vitamins.

Incorporating these nutrient-rich foods into your diet supports the biochemical processes that underpin mental health, helping to maintain a balance of neurotransmitters and hormones that regulate mood and cognitive function.

The gut-brain axis

The gut–brain axis is a complex communication network that links the digestive system and the brain. Often referred to as a 'second brain', this connection plays an important role in mental health, as the gut microbiome – composed of trillions of bacteria, viruses, and other microbes – plays a significant role in producing neurotransmitters and regulating inflammation, both of which influence mood and cognitive function. Research has shown that a healthy gut microbiome can contribute to improved mental well-being, while an unhealthy gut can increase symptoms of anxiety, depression, and other mental health issues (Firth *et al.* 2020). For example, an overgrowth of specific types of bacteria may be associated with depressive symptoms, while a depletion of other beneficial bacteria also correlates with depressive symptoms (Radjabzadeh *et al.* 2022; Valles-Colomer *et al.* 2019).

The gut–brain axis operates through various pathways, including the vagus nerve, the immune system, and the neuroendocrine system. The vagus nerve connects the brain to the gut and helps regulate internal organ functions such as digestion and heart rate. The immune system, particularly the low-grade inflammation seen in many mental health disorders, also plays a role in this connection. Additionally, the neuroendocrine system, which involves gut hormones, can influence mood and stress responses (Chakrabarti *et al.* 2022).

The relevance of the gut–brain axis lies in its impact on mood and cognitive function. Those experiencing anxiety, depression, and obsessive thoughts can benefit from improving their gut health through diet and lifestyle changes. A healthier gut can lead to more stable mood and energy levels, reducing the intensity of stress and promoting a more positive self-perception.

The key takeaway here is that to support the gut–brain axis, it's vital to adopt a comprehensive approach to improving gut health. In my clinical practice, it's rare to find someone with perfect gut health. Often, people are unaware of or accustomed to having irregular gut function. Some clients think it's normal to go to the bathroom six times per day with liquid consistency, while others think it's normal to only pass a stool once per week.

Understanding gut health can be tricky, as the causes of gut health problems vary greatly from one person to the next. I always strive to identify the root cause of digestive issues. It's important to explore all potential factors rather than just accepting a diagnosis like irritable bowel syndrome (IBS) at face value.

Improved gut health can also have a positive impact on both mental well-being and skin health. When the gut functions optimally, it enhances the body's ability to absorb essential nutrients, promoting clearer skin, healthier hair, and stronger nails. Moreover, a balanced gut microbiome can reduce inflammation, which is often linked to skin conditions such as acne and eczema (Mahmud *et al.* 2022). These aesthetic improvements can boost self-esteem and positively influence body image, contributing to an overall sense of well-being. When taking a holistic approach, addressing both mental and physical health through diet and gut health, individuals can support long-term emotional and physical well-being.

To fully support gut health, it's important to consider the following aspects:

- Removing sensitive or inflammatory foods that can harm the gut: This could be foods to which you may be allergic or sensitive. The best way to work this out is by doing an elimination diet, where you remove one potential trigger food at a time (such as gluten or dairy) for three weeks, then slowly reintroduce it while monitoring symptoms. To get accurate results, it's best to conduct this separately from other dietary changes, such as reducing ultra-processed and high-sugar foods. Otherwise, improvements in symptoms might be mistakenly attributed to removing a specific allergen when they are actually due to an overall healthier diet. However, minimizing ultra-processed and high-sugar foods remains beneficial in the long run, as these can contribute to inflammation and disrupt the gut microbiome.

- Considering possible gut infections or bacterial/fungal over-growth: Sometimes digestive issues are due to infections or an overgrowth of bacteria or fungi in the gut, such as small intes-tinal bacterial overgrowth or Candida overgrowth. Signs that this might be the case include persistent bloating, gas, diarrhoea or constipation, unexplained fatigue, sugar cravings, brain fog, or frequent yeast infections. It's important to get tested if you suspect this might be the case and take relevant action under the supervision of a professional.

- Ensure you are digesting well: The most common advice I give in regard to gut health is to chew food thoroughly. Try closing your eyes in between mouthfuls to get an idea of how much you should chew. Proper chewing aids digestion and helps the body absorb nutrients more efficiently.

- Adding in live bacteria: This can be achieved by adding fer-mented foods such as kimchi, sauerkraut, yoghurt, kefir, miso, and kombucha. These foods are rich in probiotics, which sup-port a healthy gut microbiome. There is always an option of using a multi-strain probiotic supplement as an alternative to fermented foods.

- Adding in fibre: Incorporate high-fibre foods such as fruit, veg-etables, legumes, whole grains, nuts, seeds, and oats into your diet. Studies have shown that diets rich in fibre, polyphenols, and unsaturated fats, such as the Mediterranean diet, can pro-mote a healthy gut microbiome (Edwards *et al.* 2017).

- Supporting stress levels: Managing stress is crucial for maintain-ing gut health. Techniques such as meditation, deep breathing exercises, and regular physical activity can help reduce stress. Advice for this is given later in the chapter as well as throughout this book.

If you resonate with poor digestive health, the key first step is to book an appointment with your doctor. You may also want to seek the advice of a nutritional therapist or functional medicine practitioner who can help tailor a gut health programme specifically for you. It's important to be mindful, especially for individuals with body dysmorphia, of potential risks associated with restrictive diets like elimination diets. Professional guidance ensures that you address any underlying issues and adopt strategies that are effective and safe for your individual needs. Testing can be completed to work out the root cause of your digestive issues, providing a clearer path to effective treatment and management.

Key nutrients for brain health

Supporting brain health is essential for maintaining mental well-being, especially for individuals with body dysmorphia. Proper nutrition can enhance cognitive function, stabilize mood, and reduce anxiety, all of which contribute to a healthier mindset and improved body image perception. Key nutrients play a pivotal role in neurotransmitter production, inflammation reduction, and overall brain function.

Protein

Protein is vital for producing neurotransmitters – chemicals that influence mood and cognitive function. When following a blood sugar balanced diet, you should naturally be getting enough protein. However, a general guideline is to consume about 0.8 to 1.2 grams of protein per kilogram of body weight. Protein-rich foods can support mental health and promote balanced brain chemistry. Some may find it useful to use a protein supplement such as whey protein or a vegan alternative to help hit protein targets.

B vitamins

B vitamins, including B6, B12, and folate, are critical for brain health. They play a role in neurotransmitter production and bodily processes affecting mood regulation and cognitive function. Deficiencies in these vitamins can lead to mood disturbances and cognitive issues, which can exacerbate symptoms of body dysmorphia by increasing anxiety and depression levels.

- B6 (pyridoxine): Supports serotonin and dopamine production. Sources include chicken, fish, potatoes, chickpeas, and bananas.
- B12: Maintains nerve cell health and DNA production. Found in meat, fish, dairy products, and fortified cereals.
- Folate: Important for DNA and RNA production and cell division. Found in leafy greens, legumes, nuts, and seeds.

Vitamin D

Vitamin D is crucial for maintaining mental health, especially in areas with limited sunlight exposure. Vitamin D deficiencies are linked to mood disorders, so supplementation can be beneficial, especially in the winter (Shah and Gurbani 2019). I would advise you to undergo test screening to check your levels if you are concerned about low vitamin D status.

Magnesium

Magnesium is crucial for brain health and mental well-being. It regulates neurotransmitters like serotonin, which influence mood, reduces stress by calming the nervous system, may improve sleep quality, and has anti-inflammatory properties that help protect the brain. Good sources of magnesium include leafy greens (spinach, kale), nuts and seeds (almonds, pumpkin seeds), whole grains (brown rice, quinoa), legumes (black beans, lentils), and fish (salmon, mackerel).

Omega-3 fatty acids

Omega-3 fatty acids are essential for brain health and mood regulation. They help reduce inflammation and support neurotransmitter function. Foods rich in omega-3s, such as fatty fish (salmon, mackerel) and plant-based sources (flaxseeds, chia seeds, walnuts), can significantly contribute to better mental health. If you are not a fan of fish, then perhaps consider a fish oil supplement or an algae supplement, which is a vegan alternative.

Antioxidants

Antioxidants help protect brain cells from damage by reducing oxidative stress, which is damage to cells caused by an imbalance of harmful molecules and the body's ability to neutralize them. A diet rich in antioxidants supports mental health by promoting a healthier brain. Foods high in antioxidants include berries, dark leafy greens, nuts, and seeds. The simplest way to think about adding antioxidants to your diet is to 'eat a rainbow' by including a variety of colourful fruit and vegetables on your plate.

Supplements

While I prefer a food-first approach, supplements can play a valuable role in complementing a healthy diet, particularly when it comes to supporting brain health. Ensuring balanced brain chemistry is crucial for managing symptoms of body dysmorphia, and supplements can help to address deficiencies that are difficult to correct through diet alone.

Choosing the right supplements

When selecting supplements, it is crucial to choose high-quality products from reputable brands that offer third-party testing and transparent ingredient sourcing. Additionally, always check for potential interactions with any medications you are taking and consult with a healthcare provider before starting any new supplements.

Key considerations for supplementation

- Active vs. inactive forms: Supplements come in different forms, and it's essential to choose the active forms of vitamins and minerals for better absorption and effectiveness. For instance, methylcobalamin is the active form of vitamin B12, which is more readily absorbed by the body compared to cyanocobalamin. Similarly, folate in the form of 5-methyltetrahydrofolate (5-MTHF) is more bioavailable (how easily a nutrient is absorbed and used by the body) than folic acid.

- Types of vitamins and minerals: Different forms of vitamins and minerals can have varying levels of bioavailability and effects. For example:
  - Magnesium: Magnesium glycinate is known for its calming

properties and is less likely to cause digestive issues, whereas magnesium malate is often used for energy production and muscle function.

- Iron: Ferrous sulphate is a common form of iron supplement, but ferrous bisglycinate is better absorbed and gentler on the stomach.

- Addressing deficiencies: Sometimes it is challenging to get enough of certain nutrients from food alone, especially if you have a deficiency. In such cases, supplements can provide the necessary amounts to support optimal brain health. Testing is advised to identify any specific deficiencies you might have, allowing for a more targeted approach to supplementation. Blood tests can reveal levels of vitamins like B12 and D and minerals like magnesium and iron, guiding appropriate supplementation. Working with a nutritional professional can help you understand this process with ease, as well as knowing dosages, timing, and staging of supplements.

- Supporting specific needs: Certain life stages, lifestyles, or conditions may require specific supplements. For instance, vegans might need B12 supplements, as this vitamin is primarily found in animal products. Older adults may require more vitamin D and calcium for bone health, which also supports overall well-being.

- Interaction with medications: Supplements can interact with medications, affecting their efficacy or causing adverse effects. For example, high doses of vitamin K can interfere with blood thinners like warfarin. Always consult with a healthcare provider to ensure that the supplements you take are safe and appropriate for your specific health needs and medication regimen.

Creating a personalized nutrition plan

Diets can often be too restrictive and triggering for individuals with body dysmorphia, making it essential to adopt a personalized approach to nutrition. The information provided so far in this chapter has been educational, offering insights into how a healthy diet impacts neurotransmitters, blood sugar, and hunger hormones, all aimed at covering one of the functional pillars in body dysmorphia recovery.

At this point, you may feel like there's a lot to take in, and perhaps even pressure to implement everything at once – adding specific nutrients, balancing blood sugar, adjusting your diet, and keeping up with all the recommendations. But that's not the philosophy I encourage. This is not about perfection or rigid adherence to a set of rules. It's about understanding your body, making choices that work for you, and taking things at your own pace.

Now, it's time to put this knowledge into practice. Creating a personalized nutrition plan is about finding what works for you, knowing your tolerances and triggers, and focusing on sustainability. Nourishing your body should remove obstacles to healing, not add more pressure, and shouldn't require you to push beyond your comfort zone. Below are some strategies to help you develop a long-lasting nutrition programme.

Steps to develop a nutrition plan
1. Assess your current diet

- Keep a journal: For 3 days, keep track of everything you eat, timings, and how you feel afterwards. This is the only time I advise tracking food and drink intake with body dysmorphia, as the purpose is to identify what foods make you feel good and those that don't.
- Identify nutrient gaps: Try to understand where improvements could be made in your current diet. This could involve assessing your intake of protein, fruit, and vegetables, or identifying high amounts of processed foods, sugar, caffeine, or alcohol.

2. Set realistic goals

- Break down goals: Break down your overall health goals into smaller, manageable steps. Make your goals more comprehensive than just losing fat or building muscle. Consider goals like improving energy levels, enhancing mood, reducing anxiety, and cultivating a positive relationship with food and your body.
- Assess overwhelm: Reflect on past experiences with diets. Have they failed because they were too strict or overwhelming? Aim to create a plan that feels manageable and compassionate. Maybe the best decision is not to create a programme right now and have a loose intention in your mind to eat intuitively to nourish your body.
- Flexibility: Allow room for flexibility in your plan. Understand that it's okay to have off days and that perfection is not the goal. Focus on consistent, positive changes rather than rigid adherence to a set plan.

3. Consider professional support

- A nutrition professional can provide personalized advice and help tailor a meal plan to your specific needs. If this is beyond your budget, consider online resources, community health programmes, or group workshops that offer nutritional guidance at a lower cost. Regular check-ins with a nutritionist can help you adjust your plan as needed based on your progress and any new challenges. Alternatively, join support groups or online forums where you can share experiences and receive advice from others on similar journeys. However, it may be more beneficial to employ a therapist at this time, as they can help address the emotional and psychological aspects of body dysmorphia, providing a more holistic approach to your recovery. Additionally, there are charities listed at the back of this book that offer support and resources for individuals dealing with body dysmorphia. There are also resources on low-cost or free therapy options.

4. Plan balanced, healthy meals

- Start with protein: Include a good source of protein in each meal to support neurotransmitter production.
- Incorporate healthy fats: Add some fatty fish, flaxseeds, or other healthy fats like nuts, seeds, avocados, and olive oil.
- Include a rainbow of vegetables: Aim for a variety of colours of fruit and vegetables to ensure a range of vitamins and antioxidants.
- Choose whole grains: Opt for whole grains like brown rice, quinoa, and oats to maintain stable blood sugar levels.
- Stay hydrated: Drink plenty of water throughout the day to support overall brain function.

5. Embrace mindful eating

- Enjoy your food: Focus on the flavours, textures, and aromas of your meals.
- Eat slowly: Take your time with each bite, savouring the experience.
- Pay attention to hunger and fullness cues: Listen to your body and eat when you're hungry, stopping when you feel satisfied.
- Limit phone use: Minimize distractions by avoiding phone use or other screens during meals.
- Prepare meals from scratch: Engage in the process of preparing your food, which can enhance appreciation and mindfulness.
- Enjoy meals with others: Eating with family or friends can enhance the experience and also provide emotional support.

6. Regular meals and snacks

- Consistent eating schedule: Eating at regular intervals helps maintain stable blood sugar levels and prevents overeating.
- Optional balanced snacks: For those that like to snack, choose options that combine protein, healthy fats, and fibre to keep you satisfied between meals.

7. Meal planning tips

- Batch cooking: Prepare large quantities of meals in advance to save time and ensure you have healthy options available throughout the week.
- Grocery lists: Create grocery lists based on your meal plan to help you stay organized and avoid impulse purchases.
- Flexible recipes: Use recipes that allow for substitutions based on what you have on hand to reduce stress and make cooking more enjoyable.

This approach ensures that your nutrition plan is tailored to your specific needs and preferences, supporting both your mental and physical health in a compassionate and sustainable way.

Weight loss medications

Weight loss medications such as Ozempic and Mounjaro can be prescribed to support weight management in individuals who require it for medical reasons. These medications work by reducing hunger and increasing fullness, but it's vital to use them under medical supervision. While they can help with weight loss, it's essential to focus on nourishing the body and understanding the underlying reasons for eating habits. In regards to body dysmorphia, the use of weight loss medications can be particularly complex. While they may lead to temporary physical changes, they do not address the psychological aspects of body dysmorphia. Additionally, discontinuing these medications can result in weight regain, which may exacerbate feelings of failure and body dissatisfaction.

It's also important to be aware of potential side effects and risks, as these medications are not suitable for everyone. Their long-term effects are still being studied, and their use should always be discussed with a healthcare provider.

Anyone considering weight loss medication should work closely with healthcare providers to develop a comprehensive plan that includes mental health support, aiming to build a healthier relationship with food and body image.

Addressing specific diets
Fasting

Fasting, particularly intermittent fasting, has gained popularity for its potential metabolic benefits. However, it is not recommended for everyone, especially those with a history of eating disorders or body dysmorphia. The restrictive nature of fasting can trigger unhealthy eating patterns and obsessions, potentially exacerbating body image issues. Additionally, if you deviate from fasting, you may start to demonize eating at regular times, like having breakfast, which can further impact your relationship with food. For those with body dysmorphia, the psychological impact of fasting must be carefully considered to avoid triggering negative behaviours.

Juicing

Incorporating juices into your diet can be a way to increase nutrient intake, but they should not replace whole foods. Juices, particularly those high in fruit sugars, can cause blood sugar spikes and lack the fibre essential for digestive health. Vegetable-based juices are a better option as they are lower in sugar and provide valuable nutrients. Juice cleanses, where individuals drink only juices for a day or more, can be particularly problematic. These cleanses can lead to extreme caloric restriction and reinforce unhealthy patterns, especially for those with body dysmorphia. Focusing on whole, unprocessed foods rather than relying on juices can promote better overall health and a more balanced relationship with food.

Ketogenic

The ketogenic diet is a high-fat, low-carbohydrate regimen that can lead to significant weight loss and improved mental clarity for some. However, it may not be sustainable long term and can impact on mental health due to its restrictive nature. The strict limitations of the ketogenic diet can be triggering and may lead to increased anxiety and obsessive behaviours around food. Additionally, there is a high probability of breaking the diet, which can result in feelings of failure and guilt, further exacerbating symptoms of body dysmorphia. Before embarking on this diet, it's important to understand how it can affect your mood and overall well-being, including the initial withdrawal phase that can cause tiredness and other discomforts. The diet's emphasis on drastically reducing carbohydrate intake can also alter your relationship with carbohydrates, leading you to view all carbs as bad, which can complicate your eating habits and nutritional balance. Ensure that a ketogenic diet is followed under professional supervision.

Vegan

A vegan diet, which excludes all animal products, is chosen by many for ethical reasons, including animal welfare and environmental concerns. For those that are vegan, it is crucial to ensure an adequate intake of protein, B12, iron, and omega-3 fats. Supplements may be necessary to avoid deficiencies that can negatively impact mental health. A well-planned vegan diet can support overall well-being and encourage a positive relationship with food, provided that nutritional needs are met and the diet does not become another form of restrictive eating.

Mediterranean

The Mediterranean diet emphasizes whole grains, healthy fats, lean proteins, and plenty of fruit and vegetables. Known for its balanced and sustainable approach, this diet supports mental health by providing a rich array of nutrients essential for brain function. Its less restrictive nature makes it suitable for individuals with body dysmorphia, promoting a healthy relationship with food without the stress of strict dieting rules. This is very similar to the diet approach I have outlined earlier in this chapter.

Paleo

The paleo diet focuses on consuming foods that our ancestors might have eaten, such as lean meats, fish, fruit, vegetables, nuts, and seeds, while avoiding processed foods, grains, and dairy. While this diet can encourage healthier eating patterns by emphasizing whole foods, it may be overly restrictive for some. For those with body dysmorphia, the emphasis on meat and exclusion of other food groups might not suit everyone's preferences or ethical considerations, and long-term adherence can be challenging.

Low-FODMAP

The low-FODMAP (fermentable oligosaccharides, disaccharides, monosaccharides, and polyols) diet is designed to manage the symptoms of IBS by eliminating certain carbohydrates that are hard to digest. This diet is often used short term under professional guidance to identify trigger foods, followed by a gradual reintroduction. While it can be effective for digestive health, its restrictive nature is not typically recommended for long-term use, nor does it solve the root cause of the digestive issue. Individuals with body dysmorphia should approach this diet cautiously, as the focus on food elimination can be triggering.

Macrodieting

Macrodieting involves tracking macronutrients – proteins, carbohydrates, and fats – to achieve specific body composition goals, and is often used in bodybuilding. While this method can be effective for muscle gain and fat loss, it requires meticulous tracking and weighing of food, which can become obsessive. For those with body dysmorphia, the detailed focus on food intake and body measurements can exacerbate anxiety and unhealthy preoccupations with body image. Additionally, the constant tracking can lead to losing the enjoyment of meals and social eating experiences, making eating feel like a chore rather than a pleasurable activity. While macrodieting has its purpose in professional bodybuilding and fitness, it is not necessarily needed for the average gymgoer. It's important to monitor how this diet impacts your mental health and ensure it does not become too restrictive or stressful.

Intuitive eating

Intuitive eating is a non-diet approach that encourages listening to your body's hunger and fullness cues. This approach is particularly beneficial for individuals with body dysmorphia as it promotes body positivity and self-compassion. Choosing to reject diet culture and focusing on internal cues, intuitive eating helps us develop healthier eating habits and a more balanced, stress-free approach to nutrition.

Do what is right for you

Choosing a diet that aligns with your personal health goals, preferences, and lifestyle is crucial. Always consider how a diet affects your mental and emotional well-being, not just your physical health. If you're interested in trying out a particular diet, educate yourself thoroughly about it, including its potential drawbacks. For those who have frequently experimented with various diets, it might be time to reject dieting altogether and focus on eating well. Tailoring your nutrition plan to suit your unique needs can help you develop a sustainable and positive relationship with food and your body. Put simply, if you find the right eating programme aligned to your lifestyle and individuality, you'll never have to keep restarting on Monday.

Emotional eating

Emotional eating is when we turn to food in response to our feelings instead of actual hunger. For many, emotional eating is a way to cope with stress, anxiety, boredom, sadness, or even happiness. It's common to crave comfort foods – those high in sugar, fat, and carbohydrates – because they provide a temporary sense of relief or pleasure. Over time, these patterns can become ingrained, and we might find ourselves reaching for food without realizing that it's a way to cope with our emotions. This can be especially true if we've learnt from a young age to associate food with comfort or reward.

Emotional eating can also stem from unresolved trauma or deeper emotional issues, creating an urge to eat as a way to fill an emotional void. Often, we're not fully conscious of the intense emotions we're experiencing; instead, our instinct is to numb the discomfort through eating, smoking, or mindlessly scrolling on our phones. This avoidance cycle makes it harder to break the habit of emotional eating and keeps us from facing the true source of our distress.

There are several underlying reasons why you might find yourself overeating:

- Past experiences: Unresolved issues from the past, such as trauma or emotional neglect, can drive emotional eating as a way to avoid confronting painful memories or feelings.

- Future worries: Anxiety about the future can trigger overeating as a way to temporarily soothe the stress and uncertainty, providing a fleeting sense of control.
- Not thinking about where your thoughts come from: A lack of awareness about the origins of your thoughts can keep you trapped in reactive patterns, like turning to food for comfort without recognizing the emotional triggers behind it.
- Not feeling good enough: Feelings of inadequacy and self-doubt often lead to using food as a way to cope with low self-esteem, reinforcing a cycle of emotional eating that can be difficult to break.
- Seeking escape or distraction: Food can act as a temporary escape from emotional pain, offering a quick distraction that momentarily shifts focus away from distressing feelings or situations.
- Stress: Daily pressures, work demands, relationship struggles, or financial worries can trigger overeating as a means of self-soothing or as an immediate comfort against life's challenges.
- Self-sabotage: A deep-rooted fear of change, success, or self-improvement can lead to deliberately undermining progress with food, reinforcing negative beliefs about self-worth, and making change feel impossible.

On the flip side, emotional responses can also cause undereating. Stress, anxiety, or a sense of losing control may lead some individuals to restrict food intake as a way to feel in control or as a subconscious form of self-punishment. Both overeating and undereating are often symptoms of deeper emotional struggles, reflecting how we try to manage pain or exert control over our lives through food.

Physiological reasons behind cravings

Cravings can stem from both our minds and bodies. Food often serves as a coping mechanism, providing temporary relief from negative emotions. Physiologically, stress and other emotional states can disrupt our hormone levels, such as cortisol, which increases our appetite and drives cravings for high-calorie foods. Eating these comfort foods releases dopamine, a neurotransmitter that makes us feel good, albeit temporarily.

People with naturally lower levels of dopamine may be more prone to emotional eating, as they seek to boost their mood and energy levels through food. This can create a cycle of dependency on high-sugar and high-fat foods to achieve short-term pleasure, further disrupting the balance of neurotransmitters in the brain.

Additionally, if a nutrient deficiency is a mitigating factor in a mental health disorder, it can be argued that these deficiencies are linked to experiencing more cravings. For example, low levels of magnesium, B vitamins, and omega-3 fatty acids are often associated with increased anxiety and depression, which may trigger cravings for comfort foods.

Impact of restrictive diets

Restrictive diets can intensify emotions as they create a void, depriving the body of its usual coping mechanisms and leading to heightened cravings and emotional distress. This is another reason why I am anti-diet, as these restrictive practices can exacerbate emotional eating patterns and make it harder to develop a healthy, balanced relationship with food. When you stop using food to fill an emotional void, you are often confronted with the underlying feelings and issues that were previously masked by emotional eating. This can be a challenging process, as it requires facing and addressing those emotions directly, which can feel overwhelming.

Emotional eating is complex and highly individual. Rather than adding more restrictions or trying new diets, the key is to aim for self-awareness of why you are emotionally eating in the first place and work on these underlying causes with compassion. Below are some suggestions on how you can manage emotional eating. This approach will be developed in subsequent chapters.

Strategies for identifying and managing emotional eating

- Self-awareness: Start by recognizing your emotional eating patterns. Where you find yourself craving certain foods, try to notice if there is a pattern to it and whether it is linked to when you eat, what you eat, or related to emotions you are experiencing at the time.

- Mindful eating: Practise mindfulness to help distinguish between physical hunger and emotional hunger. Focus on the sensory experience of eating, such as the taste, texture, and aroma of food, to enhance enjoyment and satisfaction.
- Developing healthy emotional outlets: Focus on developing a broad range of strategies to manage emotions, such as engaging in physical activity, learning a new skill or hobby, and practising relaxation techniques. These approaches will be discussed in more detail in the following chapters, providing you with the tools to address emotional eating and improve overall mental health.
- Balanced approach: Allow yourself to enjoy all foods occasionally without guilt. Completely restricting certain foods can lead to increased cravings and binge eating. Remember, it's okay to enjoy a biscuit or some chocolate. A balanced approach to eating allows for flexibility and enjoyment, reducing the need for restriction – and the subsequent risk of emotional eating – while maintaining a healthy relationship with food. This was especially hard for me to embody initially. I vividly remember the nostalgia I experienced from having some childhood biscuits, which gave me so much comfort and joy; but on the flip side, the voice in my head was telling me off because they were full of sugar and not in line with my diet. Instead of fully embracing the moment, I found myself torn between the pleasure of the past and the constraints of my present choices, caught in a moment of internal conflict.

Stress and its impact

Stress significantly impacts eating behaviours and can exacerbate body dysmorphia. Stress can amplify negative body image thoughts and drive emotional eating as a coping mechanism, creating a difficult cycle to break.

By recognizing how stress influences your eating behaviours, you can develop strategies to manage cravings and improve your relationship with food. This balanced approach supports both physical and mental well-being. Additionally, by addressing stress through nutritional and physiological means, you can create a more balanced approach to managing emotional eating and body dysmorphia. This foundation of support will be complemented by lifestyle strategies discussed in subsequent chapters, helping you build a holistic approach to stress reduction and overall well-being. Examples of ways to manage emotional eating include the following:

- Prioritize nutrient-rich foods: You should be aware by now of the importance of a balanced blood sugar level for optimal health. Emphasize the importance of nutrient-dense foods and use the guidelines provided in the 'Creating a personalized nutrition plan' section above to tailor your approach. Incorporate a variety of lean proteins, whole grains, fruit, and vegetables. These foods provide essential nutrients that help the body manage stress more effectively and maintain stable energy levels.
- Regular meals: Eating regular meals prevents low blood sugar levels, which can trigger stress responses and increase cravings for unhealthy foods. Maintain a consistent eating schedule to support steady energy levels.
- Mindful eating: Practising mindful eating helps you become more aware of your hunger and fullness cues. This awareness can reduce the tendency to use food as a coping mechanism for stress.
- Limit caffeine and alcohol: Caffeine and alcohol can interfere with sleep and exacerbate stress. Try to limit your intake of caffeine after 1 p.m., including sources such as coffee, tea, chocolate, cola, and energy drinks. Instead, opt for calming herbal teas or water.
- Stay hydrated: Proper hydration supports overall bodily functions and can help manage stress. Dehydration can increase cortisol levels, so aim for around 2–3 litres of fluid per day, adjusting based on your individual needs, activity level, and climate.
- Incorporate omega-3 fatty acids: Foods rich in omega-3 fatty acids can help reduce inflammation and support brain health, enhancing your resilience to stress.
- Magnesium-rich foods: Magnesium has calming effects on the nervous system. Include magnesium-rich foods to help manage stress levels. If you are opting for a magnesium supplement, I recommend using magnesium glycinate for its calming effects.

- B vitamins: B vitamins are essential for managing stress and maintaining mental health. They help convert food into energy, support the nervous system, and produce neurotransmitters that regulate mood.
- Vitamin C: This is a powerful antioxidant that helps protect the body from the harmful effects of stress by reducing oxidative damage. It also supports the immune system and aids in the production of neurotransmitters. Foods rich in vitamin C include citrus fruits, strawberries, bell peppers, broccoli, and Brussels sprouts. Together, these vitamins help maintain a balanced mood and enhance resilience to stress. When choosing a vitamin C supplement, opt for one that offers high bioavailability, such as ascorbic acid with bioflavonoids or liposomal vitamin C.
- Consider adaptogens: Incorporating adaptogens into your routine can be a valuable strategy for managing stress and enhancing overall well-being. Adaptogens such as ginseng, rhodiola, and ashwagandha help increase resilience to stress, reduce fatigue, and improve mental performance. These herbal supplements work by supporting cortisol balance and promoting a more stable stress response. They can be taken individually or as part of a supplement complex designed to bolster your body's ability to handle stress more effectively.
- Prioritize sleep: Adequate sleep is crucial for managing stress and supporting mental health. Poor sleep can increase cortisol levels and amplify feelings of anxiety and stress. Aim for 7–9 hours of quality sleep per night. Establish a consistent sleep routine, create a restful sleep environment, and avoid caffeine and electronics before bedtime to improve sleep quality.

Emotional eating involves turning to food in response to feelings rather than hunger, often driven by stress, unresolved trauma, and ingrained habits. Recognizing these triggers and addressing them with self-awareness and compassion is key. Incorporate nutrient-dense foods and balanced eating practices to support your overall well-being. As we move forward into subsequent chapters, I hope to bolster support for addressing the underlying reasons for emotional eating.

My hope in this chapter is to have provided an understanding of the complex connection between nutrition and mental health, especially in the context of body dysmorphia. It's important to remember that all the information shared is meant to guide you, not overwhelm you. Take what resonates with you and feels relevant to your personal journey.

Diet and nutrition are incredibly personal. What works for one person might not work for another. The key is to find a balanced approach to eating that supports your well-being. If something feels like even a slight inconvenience, it's more likely to be unsustainable. Your goal should be to make changes that feel natural and supportive, not restrictive or punishing.

Understanding how hunger is influenced by biology and the impact of restrictive diets, you can avoid common pitfalls that exacerbate body dysmorphia symptoms. You now possess the tools to develop a nutrition plan tailored to your unique needs and preferences, focusing on nutrient-rich foods and balanced meals, and allowing for flexibility. If you're looking for a broader perspective on nutrition and lifestyle within the LGBTQ+ community, I encourage you to explore my first book, *Naked Nutrition: An LGBTQ+ Guide to Diet and Lifestyle* (O'Shaughnessy 2022), which will be available as a new and updated edition under the title *The Queer Guide to Nutrition and Lifestyle* in 2026. Alongside practical guidance on optimizing diet, balancing fitness goals, and supporting mental health within the context of LGBTQ+ identity, it also explores key topics such as nutrition for those living with HIV, navigating the party lifestyle, sexual health, and more.

This journey isn't about perfection; it's about making sustainable, positive changes that support your overall health. There will be times when you make different choices or have moments that don't align with your intentions. Instead of seeing these moments as setbacks, view them as opportunities to learn and grow. Each experience offers valuable insights into your habits and triggers, helping you to refine your approach and make more sustainable changes.

In the upcoming chapters, we'll explore fundamental aspects that will aid in integrating these principles into your journey. Understanding the significant effects of past trauma on body dysmorphia as well as the underlying reasons behind your thought patterns are essential elements in the journey towards recovery from body dysmorphia.

CHAPTER 4

The Impact of Trauma

U NRESOLVED TRAUMA CAN CAST A LONG SHADOW OVER OUR LIVES, affecting everything from our self-esteem to our body image. For many gay individuals, this trauma often stems from early life experiences, discrimination, or rejection. But what exactly is trauma? Trauma can be a deeply distressing or disturbing experience that overwhelms an individual's ability to cope. It can be an acute event, such as a physical assault or sudden loss, or it can develop from prolonged experiences, like ongoing discrimination, bullying, or neglect. Trauma doesn't always look like what we might expect. It can be subtle and deeply personal. Many of us might not even realize that we have experienced trauma. It's important to recognize that trauma doesn't need to be loud or catastrophic to have lasting impact. It can also be a series of more subtle, cumulative experiences – those quiet, overlooked moments of rejection, shame, feeling different, or not fitting in – that silently shape how we view ourselves. These smaller, often underestimated experiences can accumulate over time, significantly affecting mental health.

Trauma diminishes a person's sense of self and affects their ability to feel a full range of emotions and experiences. These harmful experiences can quietly shape how we view ourselves, laying the groundwork for BDD to take root. This chapter will explore the impact of trauma and offer some approaches that might help you to begin the healing process.

The journey of understanding and committing to heal from trauma is a deeply personal one, fraught with challenges and revelations. As I share my insights and experiences, particularly within the context of the gay communities' lived experiences, I hope to shed light on the complex nature of trauma while offering strategies for beginning the healing and self-acceptance journey.

Body dysmorphia: the shadow of trauma

The undercurrent of trauma in body dysmorphia is deeply significant. For many of us, early experiences of bullying, rejection, and discrimination embed a firmly established belief that we are not good enough. This pervasive feeling of inadequacy is often the result of being ostracized for our true selves, with a side effect often being a hyper-focus on our bodies as a means to gain control and acceptance.

Trauma shapes our self-perception in insidious ways. The constant message from society, and sometimes even from within our own communities, is that we must conform to certain standards of beauty and behaviour to be accepted. These external pressures can become internalized, creating a relentless drive to perfect our bodies in an attempt to compensate for the shame and rejection. The body becomes a battleground for our unresolved emotional pain.

Addressing the root of trauma is vital in the recovery from body dysmorphia. Without acknowledging and beginning the journey to healing these wounds, efforts to change one's body image are often superficial and temporary. True healing requires a journey inward, to the very heart of our pain and fear. It means understanding that the issue is not really about the body at all but about the unresolved emotional pain that has been projected onto the body. Healing requires us to face the painful experiences that have shaped our self-image and to challenge the false beliefs we have internalized about our worth and appearance.

Be gentle with yourself

This chapter may be a struggle for many readers, as delving into past traumas can be incredibly painful. I hope you approach this process with gentleness and self-compassion. You might find that memories and emotions you thought were long buried come to the surface. This is a natural part of the healing process, but it can be overwhelming. Give yourself permission to take breaks, seek support, and move at your own pace.

Remember that healing is a deeply personal process, and there is no right or wrong way to go about it. The goal is not to achieve perfection but to move towards a place of greater self-acceptance and peace.

My own struggle with trauma

I never truly grasped the impact of trauma. I believed that what had happened to me was just part of life, and since it was so long ago, it couldn't possibly still affect me. I thought that by building a tough exterior, I could protect my inner child from further pain. I believed that if I appeared strong and unbreakable, I wouldn't be bullied any more, and people would accept me. What I didn't realize was how deeply trauma had influenced my behaviours and personality, shaping who I had become.

I lacked authenticity in most areas of my life. I surrounded myself with people I knew I couldn't trust and forced a smile while serving juice to guests at a retreat where I was working. Deep down, I was living a lie. The reason for this was that I never felt truly safe. My past traumas had instilled in me a constant sense of fear and distrust, making it difficult to form genuine connections or feel secure in my own skin. This lack of safety led me to adopt a façade, masking my true self in an attempt to protect myself from further pain and rejection.

As time went on, I began to realize there were traumatic events I had forgotten entirely – whether they were repressed memories or moments I blacked out in self-protection, I can't be sure. One of these was childhood sexual abuse. It wasn't something I had consciously thought about before, but through my healing journey, the memories started to surface. When I finally uncovered it, everything started to make sense. It explained why I had always felt so emotionally closed off and fearful of human beings, why I instinctively put up walls, and perhaps even why I felt more comfortable using drugs to have sex – it was easier that way, a way to dissociate from the moment. It also helped me understand why I never let anyone get too close, even when I desperately wanted connection.

The trauma I experienced as a child and young adult led me to want to degrade my body at every opportunity, sometimes even unconsciously exposing myself to risky situations. I didn't care about the side effects of using anabolic steroids because, deep down, I felt so worthless. I thought, 'How could they possibly be worse than what I've already endured?' I put myself in physically and mentally taxing situations, like afterparties (or 'chillouts' as they are more commonly called), taking all kinds of substances just to escape the pain I couldn't comprehend, but in the moment I thought I was just having fun. I even turned to sex work, seeing it as another way to degrade my body and numb the inner turmoil I couldn't face.

It felt good to take out my frustrations on my body, but I was trapped in a complex cycle of self-destruction with no end in sight. All I knew was that I was anxious, never stopping to contemplate that this may be a combination of my hormones going haywire, the excess partying, and the trauma I had experienced exacerbating my mental state. I was stuck in a cycle of wanting to look good through training and eating well, yet exhausting myself with weekend partying and then trying to save face during the week as I worked as a nutritionist.

I was both unaware of how trauma was manifesting, yet had an inkling that what lay underneath the carpet of pain was too unbearable to even approach, and I lacked the tools to even attempt to do so. Until I found my healing path, the accumulation of my trauma resulted in an extreme hyper-vigilant state and a very low threshold for stress, as well as concurrent digestive and skin issues, which I couldn't explain. On top of this, I grappled daily with the shame of having suicidal thoughts and not knowing how to reach out for help.

I'm sharing my story because I want others to understand the pervasive nature of trauma and how it can silently shape our lives, even when we think we've left it behind. Through sharing my experiences, I hope to shed light on the ways trauma can manifest – and perhaps prompt you to think about how what you have been through has shaped your own life. We often believe that our pasts don't define us, but without addressing and understanding our trauma, we can't truly move forward and fully break free from the chains of body dysmorphia.

The manifestation of trauma

Trauma is not just a psychological experience; it leaves tangible marks on the body. Its effects can be seen in chronic physical ailments, mental health challenges, and the ways we interact with the world around us. Understanding how trauma manifests in the body and mind is crucial for comprehending its widespread effects.

Trauma isn't just a fleeting experience; it accumulates over time and embeds itself in our very being. Stored in our muscles, tissues, and even at a cellular level, trauma leaves a distinct impact on both our physical and mental health. Substantial evidence supports that trauma has significant consequences that manifest in the following ways.

Physical manifestations

- Chronic pain and tension: People who have experienced trauma are more likely to suffer from chronic pain conditions. Trauma keeps the body in a constant state of heightened alertness, leading to muscle tension and pain. This persistent readiness, part of the body's 'fight or flight' defence mechanism, can wear down muscles and tissues over time, resulting in chronic pain. Studies have also found a higher prevalence of chronic pain disorders among trauma survivors (McBeth *et al.* 2001). These physical manifestations of trauma can also feed into body dysmorphia, as the chronic discomfort can heighten self-awareness of the body, amplifying insecurities and triggering obsessive behaviours. For many, the body becomes a focus of control when other aspects of life feel overwhelmingly out of reach.
- Gastrointestinal issues: Trauma and stress can significantly impact gastrointestinal health, leading to conditions like IBS. The gut–brain axis highlights how interconnected our digestive system is with our emotional state (Mayer 2011).
- Cardiovascular problems: Chronic stress from trauma can increase heart rate and blood pressure, contributing to long-term cardiovascular issues. Research has shown that post-traumatic stress disorder (PTSD) is linked with a higher risk of cardiovascular disease (Cohen, Edmondson and Kronish 2015).
- Immune system suppression: Chronic stress from trauma can suppress the immune system, making individuals more susceptible to illnesses and infections due to the continuous release of stress hormones like cortisol (Glaser and Kiecolt-Glaser 2005).

Psychological concerns

- Anxiety and depression: Trauma can lead to a persistent state of fear and helplessness, often resulting in anxiety and depression.

These conditions are frequently observed in trauma survivors (Kessler *et al.* 2013).

- PTSD: PTSD is a severe manifestation of trauma characterized by flashbacks, severe anxiety, and uncontrollable thoughts about the traumatic event. Research has shown that individuals with PTSD often have altered brain function and structure, particularly in areas associated with fear and memory (Bremner 2006).

- Cognitive impairments: Trauma can affect cognitive functions such as memory and concentration, making it challenging for survivors to focus, remember details, or complete tasks. Trauma can shrink the hippocampus (which plays a key role in memory and learning) and affect the prefrontal cortex (responsible for rational decision-making) in the brain, leading to these impairments (Bremner 2006).

- Body dysmorphia: Trauma can also contribute to the development of BDD. Research has found that those with a history of trauma were more likely to develop BDD (Didie *et al.* 2008).

- Dissociation and desensitization: Trauma can lead to dissociation, a mental process whereby a person disconnects from their thoughts, feelings, memories, or sense of identity. This can manifest as feeling detached from oneself or the world, experiencing gaps in memory, or feeling as though one is observing oneself from outside the body. Desensitization, on the other hand, involves becoming numb to emotional experiences, which can be a protective mechanism to avoid the pain of trauma. While these responses can provide temporary relief, they often interfere with daily functioning and relationships, making it challenging to fully engage with life.

The impact on the nervous system

Trauma often results in the up-regulation of the nervous system, maintaining a state of hyper-arousal. This prolonged state of alertness can lead to chronic stress and anxiety. Many people remain unaware that they are even in this heightened state, as it becomes their new baseline for 'relaxation'. Over time, the body's internal signals become so accustomed to this elevated stress level that it no longer recognizes what true calm feels like. This misalignment can make it difficult to distinguish between safety and danger. According to polyvagal theory, which explains how our nervous system processes cues of safety, trauma can disrupt this system, causing individuals to overlook red flags or warning signs in stressful situations. As a result, high-stress environments may feel 'normal' to them, while peaceful situations might feel unnerving or unfamiliar. The brain, particularly the amygdala (involved in detecting danger) and the prefrontal cortex, becomes less effective at distinguishing real threats from perceived ones, leaving one unaware of when they are in unsafe environments.

For some of us, this heightened alertness becomes addictive as our bodies grow accustomed to operating in this state of chronic stress. When finally given the opportunity to relax, they may experience panic or discomfort because their system is no longer used to calm. This paradoxical reaction occurs because relaxation feels unfamiliar and threatening. Moreover, during moments of relaxation, long-suppressed emotions and feelings may surface, which can be overwhelming and may deter someone from seeking or embracing calm environments in the future.

Trauma affects both emotional and cognitive functioning by altering brain structures. With the hippocampus often shrinking, it can make it harder to differentiate between past and present experiences. Additionally, trauma can impair the brain's ability to regulate emotions and handle stress, contributing to persistent feelings of overwhelm and distress. These changes explain why trauma often feels so all-encompassing and difficult to process.

Relationships

Trauma can significantly impact interpersonal relationships. Individuals may struggle with trust and intimacy, leading to isolation and difficulty forming healthy connections. This difficulty in relationships stems from past betrayals or hurt, making it hard to trust others and open up emotionally. The hyper-arousal state maintained by the nervous system can make things worse as individuals remain on high alert, constantly wary of potential threats. This combination of factors often results in a cycle of isolation and loneliness, further entrenching the effects of trauma on one's social life and emotional well-being.

Genetic expression

Trauma can even influence genetic expression, suggesting that its effects can be inherited and experienced at a biological level. For instance, research by Yehuda *et al.* (2016) found that descendants of Holocaust survivors had altered stress hormone profiles, predisposing them to anxiety and stress-related disorders.

Why trauma manifestations are often overlooked

Despite its significant impact, the physical manifestation of trauma is often overlooked for several reasons. The primary association of trauma with mental health issues like PTSD, anxiety, and depression can overshadow the recognition of its physical effects. This focus on mental health means that physical symptoms are often attributed to other causes and not linked back to trauma. Modern medicine frequently treats the mind and body separately, with specialists focusing on either psychological or physical health, resulting in fragmented care where the interconnectedness of trauma's effects on the body and mind is not fully addressed. There is also a general lack of awareness about how deeply trauma can affect the body, leading people to overlook that their chronic pain, digestive issues, or other physical symptoms could be rooted in unresolved trauma. Additionally, trauma is hard to measure in a lab because it is deeply personal and subjective. The effects of trauma vary widely among people, making it difficult to quantify and study in a controlled setting. Furthermore, discussing trauma and its effects can be stigmatizing, causing many to suffer in silence and preventing them from seeking help and understanding the full scope of their symptoms. Cultural attitudes that prioritize resilience and endurance may view the acknowledgement of trauma and its effects as a sign of weakness, discouraging individuals from exploring the physical manifestations of their trauma.

Specific traumas in the gay community

When we examine the subject of trauma within the gay community, we must recognize the multitude of experiences that shape the lives of many gay individuals. For many of us, subtle social rejections, microaggressions, and the constant feeling of being 'othered' can create a background of continuous stress. While often dismissed as minor, these experiences accumulate over time, affecting self-perception, contributing to internalized shame, and reinforcing body dysmorphia. These experiences are marked by deep feelings of inadequacy, internalized homophobia, and the lasting impact of the HIV/AIDS epidemic. Each of these factors contributes to a complex emotional landscape, significantly influencing mental health and overall well-being.

Shame and internalized homophobia

Shame often begins early, fuelled by societal rejection and negative attitudes towards homosexuality. This isn't just a fleeting feeling of embarrassment; it's a pervasive sense of being fundamentally flawed. Internalized homophobia compounds this by embedding society's homophobic attitudes into one's own self-view. Growing up in an environment that frequently invalidates their identity, they absorb these negative messages of rejection, leading to chronic self-criticism, low self-esteem, and a persistent sense of unworthiness.

For many, this internal struggle begins at a young age, when they first realize their feelings diverge from societal norms. The fear of rejection from family, friends, and society can create a lifelong battle with self-acceptance. This internal conflict often manifests in anxiety, depression, and other mental health issues as individuals wrestle with the parts of themselves they've been taught to despise. As discussed by Alan Downs in *The Velvet Rage* (2012), many gay men attempt to over-compensate for these feelings of inadequacy by striving for perfection in various aspects of life, such as career success, physical appearance, and material wealth. This relentless pursuit of external validation often masks entrenched feelings of shame and unworthiness. Additionally, the constant performance of heteronormative behaviours to fit into a predominantly straight world further alienates them from their true selves, keeping a cycle of emotional turmoil and disconnection going.

The impact of HIV/AIDS

The HIV/AIDS epidemic has left a lasting mark on the gay community. During the height of the crisis in the 1980s and early 1990s, the epidemic affected communities, creating an atmosphere of fear and loss. Many gay men lost friends, lovers, and mentors to AIDS, and the trauma of these losses is still felt today. The epidemic also brought intense stigma, as HIV/AIDS was heavily associated with homosexuality. This stigma compounded existing shame and isolation, creating an environment where fear and prejudice thrived.

Even with the advent of effective treatments like highly active antiretroviral therapy, which transformed HIV from a death sentence into a manageable condition, the psychological scars remain. Older gay men who lived through the worst years of the epidemic continue to carry the weight of that experience. Younger generations, while not facing the same immediate threat, still grapple with the legacy of stigma and discrimination associated with HIV. Within the community itself, the virus has sometimes been unfairly used as a marker of moral failing. This has led to 'gay-on-gay' shaming, where those with HIV may be judged and ostracized by their peers, further deepening their emotional wounds and exacerbating their sense of isolation.

The introduction of pre-exposure prophylaxis (PrEP) as a preventative measure against HIV, while revolutionary, can also serve as a constant reminder of the ongoing threat of the virus. For many, PrEP has been a lifesaver, offering a powerful tool in the fight against HIV by significantly reducing the risk of transmission. However, for some, taking PrEP daily can evoke memories of the epidemic's darkest days and the fear and stigma that accompanied it. Additionally, the emergence of other health crises, like monkeypox, can trigger similar fears and anxieties within the community. These health crises can incite more prejudice and rejection both within and outside the community.

Other specific traumas

In addition to these core issues, the gay community faces other specific traumas. Many individuals experience rejection from their families, friends, and religious communities when they come out. This rejection can lead to homelessness, especially among young people, and a sense of being utterly alone in the world. Those who cannot come out due to fear of these consequences endure a constant state of hiding and anxiety, which can severely impact their mental health. The fear of being discovered and the necessity to conceal one's true identity can lead to chronic stress, depression, and a permeating sense of isolation.

Physical and verbal assaults, bullying in schools, and hate crimes are tragically common, leaving both physical and emotional scars that can last a lifetime. Even witnessing these incidents being reported in the media can be deeply distressing, reinforcing feelings of vulnerability and fear within the community. Despite advances in legal rights, discrimination remains a pervasive issue in areas including the workplace, housing, and healthcare. This ongoing struggle for equal treatment is exhausting and dehumanizing, as individuals continuously advocate for their rights and navigate hostile environments. Seeking help for mental health issues is also fraught with challenges, as the stigma surrounding both mental health and LGBTQ+ identities can make it difficult to find supportive and understanding care.

Intersectionality also plays a significant role in compounding these traumas. Intersecting identities, such as ethnicity and socioeconomic status, can amplify the challenges faced by gay people. For example, a person of colour may face both racism and homophobia, leading to even greater levels of stress and marginalization. Similarly, trans individuals – especially those who are also gay – may experience transphobia alongside homophobia, making it even more difficult to find safe spaces and support. Additionally, those from lower socioeconomic backgrounds may face additional stressors such as financial instability and limited access to healthcare, further complicating their trauma. Recognizing these intersections is crucial for a comprehensive understanding of how trauma impacts different members of the community, not just by increasing the burden but also by how it is experienced, internalized, and processed.

All these factors can result in body dysmorphia within the gay community. The intense feelings of inadequacy and shame from these traumas can lead individuals to fixate on achieving an ideal body image as a coping mechanism. Understanding the layers of trauma within the gay community is the first step towards harbouring self-awareness about the impact of these challenges, particularly in relation to body dysmorphia. Recognizing the historical impact of various factors unique to the gay community helps to illuminate how they have shaped mental health and overall well-being. Even if some of these issues no longer overtly affect us, their historical impact continues to resonate within the community as a collective trauma.

The pain in feeling the pain: why we bury our trauma

Facing trauma can be an incredibly painful and daunting process, which is why many people tend to avoid it. The very thought of revisiting traumatic experiences can evoke intense emotions such as anxiety, fear, sadness, and anger. Confronting these feelings requires a level of vulnerability and courage that can be overwhelming. Consequently, many individuals choose to bury their trauma, sweeping it under the carpet in the hope that it will fade away on its own. However, burying trauma doesn't make it disappear; it merely intensifies its impact over time. Unresolved pain and emotional turmoil manifest in various destructive ways, often surfacing when least expected. This can lead to a range of issues, including chronic stress, anxiety, and depression. It can also result in unhealthy coping mechanisms like substance use and self-harm, as well as personality changes such as increased irritability and difficulty trusting others. Trauma can substantially impact one's sense of identity. Some may struggle with self-concept and personal identity, feeling disconnected from their true selves. This can lead to a constant search for identity and belonging, often resulting in further emotional distress. The longer trauma is ignored, the more deeply it embeds itself in the psyche, influencing behaviour and overall well-being in increasingly harmful ways.

Avoidance and coping mechanisms

To cope with the overwhelming feelings that trauma brings, many resort to avoidance mechanisms – a specific type of coping strategy. These can include excessive control over body image, substance use, and compulsive behaviours. For example, using drugs and alcohol serves as a temporary escape from the pain but often leads to addiction and further mental health issues. Similarly, excessive control over body image can manifest in eating disorders or obsessive fitness routines as individuals attempt to gain control in an unmanageable life.

Compulsive engagement in work, hobbies, or social activities can distract from painful emotions and thoughts. Focusing excessively on the needs and problems of others can serve as a distraction from one's own trauma. As a defence mechanism, some may emotionally numb themselves to cope with trauma. This numbing can prevent them from fully experiencing both negative and positive emotions, leading to a diminished capacity for joy and connection. While these avoidance strategies can provide temporary relief, they often prevent individuals from addressing the root causes of their trauma, leading to a cycle of avoidance and prolonged suffering.

Psychological impacts of avoidance

The avoidance of trauma can significantly impact psychological well-being. Increased anxiety, dissociation, and depression are common outcomes. Dissociation, in particular, can make someone feel disconnected from their own bodies and emotions, further complicating the healing process. This disconnection can contribute to body dysmorphia, they may struggle to perceive their bodies accurately, leading to obsessive and distorted views of their physical appearance. Anxiety and depression often accompany these feelings, contributing to a sense of hopelessness and helplessness. This emotional turmoil makes it even more challenging to confront the root causes of these feelings, as the person becomes trapped in a cycle of avoidance and self-criticism.

Avoidance behaviours can erode one's sense of self-worth and self-efficacy. The constant effort to suppress and ignore traumatic memories and emotions can lead to diminished capacity for joy and a reduced ability to form and maintain healthy relationships. Trauma can be passed down through generations, affecting not just those who directly experienced it but also their descendants. This concept of intergenerational trauma highlights how unresolved pain can perpetuate cycles of suffering within families and communities. Over time, the cumulative effect of these avoidance strategies can result in chronic mental health issues, physical health problems, and a significantly impaired quality of life. Recognizing and addressing these interconnected issues is crucial for breaking the cycle and beginning the healing process.

The subtle influences of trauma

Trauma doesn't always manifest in overt ways; it can subtly influence one's worldview and actions in ways that are often difficult to recognize. For instance, an unconscious reluctance to let others get close may stem from past traumatic experiences. This self-protective behaviour, while initially a defence mechanism, can lead to prolonged isolation and difficulty forming meaningful relationships. The fear of vulnerability and potential hurt creates a barrier to intimacy, causing individuals to miss out on deep, supportive connections.

Additionally, there might be a tendency to overly rationalize someone's hurtful behaviour, dismissing one's own emotional response in the process. This rationalization often comes from a desire to maintain harmony or avoid conflict, but it can also result in neglecting one's own needs and feelings. Over time, this pattern can erode self-esteem and reinforce feelings of unworthiness.

Trauma can also influence daily decision-making and interactions in more subtle ways. For example, someone who has experienced trauma may avoid certain situations or people that remind them of their past pain, limiting their social and professional opportunities. They may also develop perfectionistic tendencies, believing that by being flawless, they can avoid criticism and rejection.

As discussed above, the impact of trauma can extend to causing physical health problems. Chronic stress from unresolved trauma can lead to a range of health issues, including insomnia, headaches, gastrointestinal problems, and a weakened immune system. These physical symptoms often perpetuate the cycle of trauma, as a person may feel increasingly helpless and out of control, and the ongoing health issues can add to their emotional burden.

Disrespecting the body as a result of trauma

When someone faces overwhelming trauma, they often turn to self-destructive behaviours to manage their unbearable feelings. Substances like drugs and alcohol may initially provide a temporary escape from pain and help individuals feel relaxed or comfortable in certain situations. However, these substances lower inhibitions, potentially leading to risky behaviours and poor decisions. This can result in dangerous situations, further trauma, and strained relationships.

Substance use takes a significant toll on the body. Some may neglect basic self-care, resulting in disrupted sleep patterns and poor nutrition. The strain on the body from not sleeping or eating properly can exacerbate both physical and mental health issues, leading to a downward spiral. The cycle of substance use can quickly escalate into addiction, worsening overall health and perpetuating the cycle of trauma. While the occasional party or social gathering isn't inherently harmful, it's the habitual use of substances as a coping mechanism that can lead to severe consequences and further entrench the impacts of trauma.

Extreme dieting and obsessive control over body image are also common ways people try to cope. These behaviours represent attempts to gain control in a life that feels chaotic and unmanageable. Unfortunately, these practices can lead to severe physical health issues, such as malnutrition, hormonal imbalances, and eating disorders like anorexia or bulimia. The relentless pursuit of an ideal body image can erode self-esteem, deepening the cycle of self-criticism and dissatisfaction.

Neglecting self-care is another response to trauma. Individuals might avoid basic self-care routines, such as proper nutrition, exercise, and hygiene, reflecting their internal turmoil and feelings of worthlessness. This neglect can cause physical health to deteriorate, creating a feedback loop where poor health exacerbates emotional distress.

Additionally, self-harm is a direct and extreme form of self-destructive behaviour. Acts such as cutting, burning, or hitting oneself are ways to externalize internal pain, providing a temporary sense of relief. However, these actions carry significant risks of infection, permanent injury, and even accidental death. Self-harm deepens the emotional scars of trauma, reinforcing negative self-perceptions and feelings of hopelessness.

The impact of these self-destructive behaviours extends beyond physical health. They strain relationships, disrupt daily functioning, and impair one's ability to achieve personal and professional goals. Addressing these behaviours is essential for recovery, requiring a compassionate and comprehensive approach that includes therapy, support groups, and lifestyle changes, which will be discussed more in this chapter and subsequent chapters.

Understanding why we bury our trauma is crucial for beginning the journey towards healing. It is essential to understand the ways and reasons why we avoid our pain and the psychological toll of leaving our trauma unresolved. Healing is incredibly challenging, but I'm someone who can vouch for it being a deeply rewarding process. This process requires patience and persistence, as well as a commitment to self-care and self-compassion. Ultimately, healing from trauma is not just about overcoming past pain but also about embracing the possibility of a brighter, healthier future. With the right support and resources, individuals can move towards a more balanced and fulfilling life, leading to resilience and hope along the way.

Anger

Anger is a powerful and often misunderstood emotion. When we're unable to express it in healthy ways, it can build up inside, affecting our thoughts, behaviours, and physical well-being. For many, anger may stem from experiences of being wronged, ignored, or mistreated, but cultural and social pressures often discourage us from showing it openly. Instead of being released, anger gets internalized and may resurface in other ways.

When anger is suppressed for too long, it can manifest in various unhealthy coping mechanisms. Growing up in environments where expressing emotions – particularly anger – is discouraged or punished, many learn to bottle up their feelings rather than release them healthily. This is especially true for those who have faced chronic rejection, bullying, or other forms of emotional distress. The inability to express anger, or even recognize it, can lead to an intense focus on areas of life where control seems possible. This may manifest as control over work, relationships, or food, but for many, especially those struggling with body dysmorphia, this anger can be directed towards the body.

Rather than surfacing as obvious rage, this anger is often displaced onto the body. It can show up as an obsession with perfection, excessive exercise, or extreme dieting. Controlling the body may feel like a way to regain power in areas where people otherwise feel powerless – whether in social, familial, or personal spheres. The body becomes an easy target, where unresolved emotions are acted out, providing a sense of control amidst deeper, and often unconscious, emotional turmoil.

Understanding this dynamic is key to healing. Addressing these feelings in healthier ways – whether through therapy, creative expression, or physical activities that don't harm the body – can help release the emotional tension that fuels body control. This process ultimately leads to a more compassionate and balanced relationship with oneself.

The willingness to heal

Healing from trauma is a significant and often challenging journey that requires a conscious decision and a strong willingness to face the pain. It starts with acknowledging that what happened to you was unjust and unacceptable. This recognition is crucial because it validates your experiences and sets the stage for healing. Understanding the injustice of trauma is important, as it often underpins the ruminations and emotional turmoil that survivors experience. Recognizing this injustice allows you to begin processing the hurt and betrayal, laying the groundwork for genuine recovery and self-compassion.

Moving out of your comfort zone

Trauma can make us so accustomed to a certain way of being that we forget who we really are. Moving out of our comfort zone is essential for healing and requires us to embrace vulnerability. Opening yourself up to feel and express your emotions requires immense courage, especially when facing past traumas. Vulnerability is not a sign of weakness but a testament to your strength and willingness to confront difficult experiences. It allows for a deeper connection with yourself and creates space for healing and growth, breaking down the barriers built by trauma and rediscovering your true authentic self.

Equally important is being honest with yourself about how trauma is impacting your life. Trauma can affect your thoughts, behaviours, and physical health in ways that might not be immediately obvious. For example, it's crucial to take a moment and ask yourself why you might be experiencing body dysmorphia. What past experiences could be influencing your current self-perception? Is there a history of criticism, rejection, or other traumatic events that might be contributing to your distorted view of your body? How is body dysmorphia manifesting for you? Perhaps take a moment to journal your thoughts, allowing the pen to flow freely and capture whatever comes to mind.

Acknowledging these connections can help you better understand the full impact of your experiences and address the underlying issues. This honesty is a vital step towards healing, as it helps you identify harmful patterns and start making changes that promote well-being. Without this fundamental acknowledgement and self-awareness, the healing process can be hindered, as unresolved pain and lack of validation continue to fuel emotional distress and self-doubt. Facing these difficult questions and recognizing the trauma behind your body dysmorphia, you can begin to dismantle the negative beliefs and start moving towards a healthier self-image and better overall well-being.

Understanding the stages of healing

Healing from trauma involves several stages that help in processing and overcoming the past:

- Acknowledgement and acceptance: Recognizing the trauma and its impact is the first step. This involves accepting that the trauma happened and acknowledging its effects on your life.
- Processing and expression: Allowing yourself to express your emotions, whether through talking, writing, or creative outlets, is crucial for processing the trauma. This stage involves working through distressing memories in a safe and controlled environment, often with the support of a therapist.
- Rebuilding and growth: This stage involves integrating the trauma into your life in a healthy way, finding new meaning, and rebuilding your sense of self. It includes developing healthy coping mechanisms and emotional regulation skills to manage intense emotions and create stability.

Asking for help: a big step towards healing

Asking for help is a vital step in the healing process, especially when dealing with body dysmorphia and trauma. Showing vulnerability and a willingness to trust others can be daunting. Many of us in the gay community develop hyper-independence, feeling the need to manage everything on our own due to past experiences of being let down, betrayed, or rejected. This self-reliance can be a barrier to healing, as it prevents healing beyond your own consciousness. Seeking help from professionals is essential to breaking the pattern and starting the bumpy road to recovery.

If you find yourself hesitant to seek help, it might be beneficial to ask yourself why. Reflect on the underlying reasons behind your reluctance. Are there specific experiences that have led you to believe that you must handle everything on your own? Do you fear judgement, rejection, or appearing weak? Understanding the roots of your resistance can be the first step in overcoming it. By acknowledging these fears and insecurities, you open up the possibility of challenging them and making room for trust and support in your healing journey.

Therapeutic approaches

Creating a safe environment for healing by understanding the widespread impact of trauma is essential. Choosing a therapist with whom you feel comfortable and compatible and selecting a modality that resonates with you can significantly enhance the effectiveness of your treatment. Some therapeutic approaches are listed below.

- Cognitive-behavioural therapy: CBT helps in changing negative thought patterns that can arise from trauma and body dysmorphia. Identifying and challenging these thoughts allows individuals to develop healthier ways of thinking and responding to their experiences.
- Eye movement desensitization and reprocessing: EMDR is effective in reprocessing traumatic memories, helping individuals to integrate these memories in a way that reduces their emotional impact. This technique involves guided eye movements that facilitate the processing of distressing memories.
- Body-centred psychotherapy: Body-centred psychotherapy focuses on the physical sensations associated with trauma, recognizing that trauma can be stored in the body as well as the mind. This approach is particularly beneficial for those with body dysmorphia, as it helps reconnect the individual with their body in a healthy way.
- Psychedelics: Substances such as ayahuasca and psilocybin have shown potential in facilitating deep emotional and

psychological healing. They work by affecting the brain's default mode network (DMN), which is involved in self-referential thoughts and the sense of self. By temporarily 'parking the ego', psychedelics disrupt the usual patterns of the DMN, allowing for new perspectives and healing insights. This can lead to significant emotional breakthroughs and a deeper understanding of oneself. It's important to note that in many countries, the use of psychedelics is illegal. If you are considering a retreat or therapy involving psychedelics, ensure that it is conducted in an authentic, safe, and legal environment. This often involves seeking out trained professionals, including qualified therapists and reputable shamans, who are experienced in guiding these sessions responsibly.

Psychedelics have been pivotal in my healing, but they should be approached with caution. Embarking on a retreat means surrendering to what plant medicine brings up. This involves letting go of control and trusting that whatever surfaces is paramount to your healing. Sometimes this means sitting with your pain, learning another side of the story, and understanding your trauma from a forgiveness perspective. It's essential to approach this journey with an open mind and a supportive environment for integration, guided by experienced professionals who can help you navigate the complexities of the experience safely. There are also some contraindications for certain medical conditions and medications, so it is important to consult with a healthcare professional to ensure safety and suitability before embarking on this journey.

- Breathwork: Breathwork can achieve similar transformative effects as psychedelics by using controlled breathing techniques to access deep emotional and psychological states. Different types of breathwork, such as conscious connected breathing, holotropic breathwork, and transformational breath, can help release stored trauma and create a sense of calm and connection to the body. The benefits of using breath as a vehicle to facilitate healing are numerous: it is legal, convenient, and allows you to maintain a sense of control – stopping if it gets too intense. Additionally, breathwork offers the advantage of being incorporated into a regular practice, providing ongoing support and resilience-building. It's important to work with a trained breathwork facilitator who can help navigate your breath healing journey.

Whatever modality you choose, it's important to be gentle and ease into it, allowing yourself time to adjust and ensuring you feel safe and supported throughout the process. Each healing journey is unique, and pushing too hard or too fast can lead to overwhelm and hinder progress. Starting slowly and respecting your own boundaries helps build a solid foundation for deeper work.

Complementary therapies

In addition to traditional therapeutic approaches, complementary therapies such as acupuncture, massage therapy, and emotional freedom technique (EFT) can also play a significant role in healing from trauma. Acupuncture, for instance, can help regulate the body's energy flow and reduce stress, while massage therapy can release physical tension and promote relaxation. EFT, also known as tapping, involves using specific points on the body to release emotional blockages and reduce stress, helping individuals process difficult emotions. These are just some examples of therapies that can be excellent adjuncts to your primary treatment plan, providing additional tools to support your healing process.

Calming the nervous system

Calming the nervous system is a fundamental aspect of healing from trauma. When the nervous system is in a state of hyper-arousal, it can be difficult to process emotions and engage in therapeutic work effectively. Here are some techniques to help soothe the nervous system.

- Deep breathing: Engaging in deep, diaphragmatic breathing can activate the parasympathetic nervous system, promoting relaxation. Try inhaling deeply through your nose for a count of four, holding for a count of four, and exhaling slowly through your mouth for a count of six. Repeat this cycle several times until you feel calmer. If you're particularly anxious, try doing this lying on your front, which can help you breathe deep into your abdomen.

- Progressive muscle relaxation: This technique involves tensing and then slowly releasing each muscle group in the body, starting from your toes and working up to your head. This practice helps to release physical tension and promotes a sense of overall relaxation. Another technique is using a guided meditation such as yoga nidra.

- Grounding exercises: Grounding techniques can help bring your focus back to the present moment and reduce feelings of anxiety. A simple grounding exercise is sitting or lying down, closing your eyes, and imagining your hands and feet growing roots like a tree, going deeper and deeper into the earth's core, anchoring you to the earth as you breathe deeply.

- Mindfulness meditation: Practising mindfulness involves focusing on the present moment without judgement. One effective mindfulness exercise is the '5-4-3-2-1' technique: identify five things you can see, four things you can touch, three things you can hear, two things you can smell, and one thing you can taste. This exercise helps ground you in the present moment and reduces anxiety.

- Nature and movement: Spending time in nature and engaging in gentle physical activity can significantly reduce stress levels. Activities like walking, gardening, or simply sitting outdoors can provide a calming effect on the nervous system. Try to do this without scrolling on your phone because this can excite the nervous system.

- Self-soothing techniques: Find activities that personally bring you comfort and relaxation, such as listening to soothing music, taking a warm bath with Epsom salts, reading a book, or engaging in creative activities like drawing or knitting.

- Self-touch and affirmations: Speaking to yourself with warmth and compassion can help shift negative self-perceptions and create a deeper sense of safety within your own body. Try placing your hands on your heart or gently stroking your arms, shoulders, or legs while repeating affirmations like, 'I love myself,' 'I am safe,' or 'My body is worthy of kindness.' Your body listens to what you say about it. If you speak to yourself with criticism and negativity, your nervous system stays in a heightened state of stress. But when you speak with kindness and reassurance, your body begins to feel safe and supported.

In addition to these techniques, consider removing or limiting factors from your lifestyle that may overstimulate your nervous system:

- Caffeine: Stimulants like caffeine can keep the body in a state of heightened alertness, making it harder to relax and calm the nervous system. Reducing or eliminating caffeine intake can help promote relaxation.
- Sugar: High-sugar intake can cause energy spikes and crashes, which can contribute to feelings of anxiety and irritability. Reducing sugar consumption can help maintain a more stable mood.
- Alcohol and drugs: These substances can alter your mood and nervous system function, often leading to increased anxiety and emotional instability. Minimizing or avoiding alcohol and recreational drugs can support a calmer nervous system.
- Excessive screen time: Overstimulation from electronic devices can keep the nervous system in a heightened state of alertness. Limiting screen time, especially before bed, can help create a more restful environment for your nervous system to recover.
- Excessive exercise: Overexerting yourself through excessive exercise can also keep your body in a state of heightened alertness and stress. Finding a balance in physical activity is essential for calming the nervous system. This will be discussed in more detail in Chapter 7.

You might find yourself resistant to trying these exercises and making these changes, as calming your nervous system might not feel comfortable or natural at first. When your system is used to being on high alert, the idea of calming down can feel unfamiliar and even challenging. However, I encourage you to try them consistently; over time, your body and mind will become more accustomed to feeling calm, especially as you gradually notice the benefits.

Rebuilding from trauma

Healing from trauma can be a bumpy journey, but the benefits are far-reaching. When you address trauma head-on, you open the door to recovery, allowing growth, resilience, and a deeper understanding of yourself. It's important to understand that healing is not about erasing the past but integrating it into your understanding of who you are. This process involves recognizing the strength you've built through your experiences, breaking free from negative patterns, and living a more authentic life. This includes creating a supportive environment to heal from body dysmorphia.

Understanding that trauma is a part of you and not something to be avoided is essential. This acceptance allows for a more integrated and holistic healing process. When acknowledging trauma's impact, you can begin to recognize the strength and resilience you have developed through these experiences. The healing journey isn't about erasing the past but about incorporating it into a fuller understanding of yourself. Embracing your trauma helps you move forward with a sense of completeness and authenticity, acknowledging that every part of your journey has contributed to who you are today.

The journey of healing from trauma is often filled with difficult moments and setbacks. It's important to acknowledge that the path to recovery is not a straight line but a winding road with its share of challenges. There will be moments of progress and triumph, but also times of struggle and regression. Setbacks can feel discouraging, but they are a natural part of the process. Each step back provides an opportunity to learn and grow, gaining a deeper understanding of yourself and your experiences.

Healing, however, involves commitment and being honest with yourself about the difficulties you face. The mind often resists this, which is something we will explore in the next chapter. Embracing these difficult moments with patience and compassion is crucial. Healing is like learning a language; it takes time, patience, and persistence. Staying committed, even when it feels tough, is what allows progress to unfold. Healing from trauma involves learning a new way of being. It is a long-term investment in your mental, emotional, and physical well-being, bringing a profound sense of inner strength.

Having a strong support network is essential for healing. Whether through friends, family, or support groups, having people who understand and validate your experiences can make a significant difference. Building these connections provides emotional support and practical assistance, helping you navigate the complexities of your healing journey. This topic is covered more in Chapter 9.

While healing can be challenging and non-linear, it brings significant benefits. It builds inner strength and resilience, making you better equipped to handle future challenges. Addressing trauma can lead to significant reductions in anxiety, depression, and other mental health issues, improving overall mental health. Healing also allows for healthier relationships by enhancing your ability to trust and connect with others. Additionally, reducing the chronic stress associated with trauma can lead to better overall physical health. Ultimately, healing creates an understanding and acceptance of yourself, leading to a more fulfilling and authentic life. As a result of working through your trauma, you naturally feel safer and more grounded in your body, eventually reaching a point where you view yourself in a more positive light and perhaps allow yourself to be loved (scary, I know). Just engaging with this chapter with an open mind, the process has already started, and you should be proud of your willingness to heal.

CHAPTER 5

Rebuilding Your Mindset

BECOMING AWARE OF YOUR THOUGHT PATTERNS IS FUNDAMENTAL for overcoming body dysmorphia. The way we perceive ourselves can either hinder or facilitate our healing journey. Often, those with body dysmorphia are their own harshest critics, constantly scrutinizing perceived flaws and inadequacies and feeling full of self-doubt. This relentless self-criticism creates a toxic mental environment, making it difficult to break free from the cycle of negative self-perception.

Understanding the power of mindset allows us to recognize that our thoughts are not fixed truths but can be reshaped and reframed. This shift is about moving from a mindset of judgement to one of understanding and kindness towards oneself. Our inner dialogue can either tear us down or lift us up. For example, instead of saying, 'I'll never be good enough,' try reframing it to, 'I'm learning and growing every day.' This small shift in language can gradually reshape how we view ourselves. Shifting from self-criticism to embracing self-compassion involves treating ourselves with the same empathy and care we would offer a close friend. Cultivating this kinder inner dialogue, we can begin to soften the harshness we direct towards ourselves, gradually building the foundations for a more supportive and encouraging mindset. I know, it's easier said than done!

At the height of my own struggles with body dysmorphia, my mindset was my greatest adversary. Every time I passed a mirror, I found myself locked in a battle with my reflection, obsessively scrutinizing what was looking back at me. It was even worse when I weighed myself and the result wasn't what I expected it to be, leading to clouded thinking, restricting food more, and focusing on measures I knew weren't good for me deep down. These behaviours were unconscious and intensified by stress, bad news, or vulnerability. The negative tone set the mood for the entire day and made even the simplest tasks overwhelming because I was fixated on my body image.

It took a while, but I learnt not to be hooked on every thought. They were impulses from ingrained beliefs, shaped by years of societal pressure, trauma, and personal insecurities. As I began to shift my mindset, I noticed changes extending beyond my perception of my body. I became more self-aware of my thoughts and behaviours, learning to question why I think the way I do. I realized how incredibly hard I had been on myself, often as a way to shield myself from further trauma. This was definitely not an overnight change but a gradual process of letting go of old beliefs and embracing healthier ones.

My relationships improved as I became less critical and more empathetic, allowing me to build stronger, more authentic connections with those around me. In my professional life, the impact was equally significant. My relentless self-criticism had often left me feeling inadequate and paralysed by the fear of making mistakes. Embracing a new mindset enabled me to approach my work with greater confidence and resilience. I became more open to feedback and willing to take risks, understanding that failure was part of the learning process. This change not only enhanced my productivity but also made my work more fulfilling while expanding my view on what health and well-being truly meant. I found a renewed motivation to work hard, driven by a healthier and more balanced and authentic perspective, ultimately leading to writing this book.

Changing my mindset transformed my entire worldview. It helped me break free from continuous self-doubt and adopt a more balanced and accepting approach to life. This is something I have to work on every day, and I still find myself getting drawn to negative thoughts and feelings, especially around my body. I view setbacks as part of the learning process. When negative thoughts resurface, I've learnt to ask what emotion is causing this thought, sit with it, and take a step back, adopting a bird's eye view to gain perspective. As I share my journey, I hope to show the importance of working on your mindset as part of your recovery from body dysmorphia.

This chapter addresses many of the core mindset challenges that accompany body dysmorphia. Changing these ingrained beliefs about how we see the world and ourselves is one of the hardest things to achieve. These beliefs are often learnt behaviours that developed as survival mechanisms, making the shift to a healthier mindset both crucial and challenging. When we focus on this transformation, we lay the groundwork for overcoming deeply entrenched patterns of self-criticism and cultivating a more compassionate and supportive internal dialogue.

This chapter may provoke and challenge you as it pushes you to confront and question long-held beliefs and behaviours. It encourages you to examine the roots of your self-perception and to embrace new ways of thinking. This process can be uncomfortable, but it is a necessary step towards healing and developing a healthier, more supportive relationship with yourself. After reading through this chapter, you may want to revisit sections of it that are particularly relevant to your personal journey. The exercises and insights provided are designed to be practical tools that can be returned to whenever you need reinforcement in your mindset shift.

Mindfulness and present moment awareness

Mindfulness, the practice of staying present and fully engaging with the current moment, can be a significant tool in recovery. It can aid self-awareness, calm us down, and allow us to break free from negative thought patterns, particularly those related to our bodies.

Often, we get caught up in the busyness of life, rushing to the next task. Many of us spend hours on our phones accumulating screen time and constantly multitasking. This constant engagement can mean we are often living more in our heads than feeling embodied. Mindfulness helps us reconnect with our bodies as well as helping to create a deeper sense of peace and self-acceptance. It helps us observe our emotions without being overwhelmed by them, enabling us to respond more thoughtfully. The benefits of mindfulness also extend to physical health, as it has been shown to improve sleep, reduce chronic pain, and lower blood pressure (Loucks *et al.* 2023; Rosenzweig *et al.* 2010; Rusch *et al.* 2019).

Being present means fully engaging with whatever we are doing at the moment, whether it's eating, walking, working, or simply breathing.

It involves focusing our attention on the here and now rather than being preoccupied with the past or worrying about the future. This practice can help reduce stress, improve concentration, and enhance our overall sense of well-being. Developing a mindful awareness of our thoughts, especially during these moments, we can start to recognize when our self-talk turns critical or harsh. This awareness allows us to gently shift towards more compassionate and supportive inner dialogue. This practice can help reduce stress, improve concentration, and enhance our overall sense of well-being.

Techniques for mindfulness

- Breathing exercises: Simple breathing techniques can anchor us in the present moment. Try focusing on your breath, noticing each inhalation and exhalation, and gently bringing your attention back whenever it wanders.
- Mindful observation: Take a moment to observe your surroundings with all your senses. Notice the colours, shapes, sounds, and textures around you. This practice can ground you in the present and encourage a sense of appreciation for your environment.
- Body scan meditation: This involves closing your eyes in a comfortable space and paying attention to different parts of your body, from your toes to the top of your head. Notice any sensations, tension, or discomfort, and breathe into those areas to release any stress.
- Mindful walking: Engage in walking with full awareness of each step. Feel the ground beneath your feet, the movement of your body, and the rhythm of your breath. This practice can transform a simple walk into a meditative experience.
- Roots exercise: Imagine yourself as a tree, with roots extending from the soles of your feet deep into the ground. With each breath, allow the roots to grow, penetrating

the core of the earth. Pause and feel the stability and support from these roots, grounding you firmly in the present moment. This visualization can help you feel more connected and centred.

Incorporating mindfulness into daily life

Mindfulness doesn't have to be limited to formal meditation sessions; it can be seamlessly integrated into everyday activities. For instance, when eating, pay attention to the taste, texture, and aroma of your food, eating slowly and savouring each bite. When conversing with others, focus entirely on the speaker, listening without planning your response or getting distracted. Likewise, approach tasks at work with single-minded focus, avoiding multitasking and dedicating your complete attention to each activity. This takes practice, and it helps to set your phone to 'Do Not Disturb'.

Incorporating mindfulness into our daily lives helps us connect more deeply with ourselves and our surroundings. Staying present and aware helps us handle life's challenges more effectively and achieve a more balanced perspective, as well as encouraging a compassionate and non-judgemental relationship with our body.

Reflexivity and self-awareness

To truly understand ourselves, we must consider the practice of reflexivity. Reflexivity is the process of examining our own thoughts, emotions, and behaviours to gain a deeper understanding of ourselves. This self-examination is not just about identifying what we think and feel but also understanding why we think and feel that way. Reflexivity invites us to look beyond the surface and question the underlying beliefs and experiences that shape our perception. It's about becoming aware of the automatic thoughts that run through our minds and understanding their origins and impacts.

Reflexivity has been a crucial tool for me, one which I still use to this very day. It helps you shift from just accepting that you struggle with body dysmorphia to questioning why you do. It allows you to become conscious that negative thoughts and emotions are deeply tied to past experiences and ingrained beliefs. By examining these thoughts and feelings, you can begin to uncover patterns – how stress would amplify self-critical thoughts or how certain situations would trigger past insecurities. This understanding is the first step towards breaking free from these automatic self-critical responses that can easily take over.

Building on the foundation of reflexivity, self-awareness involves a deeper understanding of our internal processes, recognizing how our thoughts, emotions, and behaviours are interconnected. It means being conscious of our triggers, our strengths, and our areas for growth. Self-awareness allows us to identify patterns in our thinking and behaviour that contribute to our body dysmorphia and our mental health.

Developing self-awareness can be challenging, especially when we are accustomed to ignoring or suppressing our emotions. However, it is essential for breaking free from negative thought patterns and cultivating a more compassionate relationship with ourselves. By becoming more self-aware, we can start to make intentional changes in our lives that support our healing journey and can help us gain insights into the underlying causes of body dysmorphia.

Consider a scenario where you are in the gym locker room and notice someone with a physique that you perceive as 'better' than yours. This observation may trigger negative thoughts about your own body, leading you to scrutinize your body and feel anxious all day. With self-awareness, you can recognize that these environments are triggers for you and start to understand the underlying emotions, such as fear of inadequacy or not measuring up. This awareness allows you to know which environments may trigger you and when to practise self-soothing, reminding yourself of your strengths, goals, and progress. Journaling is a great tool to help you reflect on where negative thoughts are triggered and understand the circumstances and emotions involved.

Reflexivity allows you to step back and view your thoughts and emotions from a distance, giving you the space to respond rather than react. It is integral to understanding the intricate relationship between our mental state and overall health. It empowers individuals to consider factors like trauma, ego state, and control in their health journey, ensuring a comprehensive approach to wellness. Reflexivity is not just about self-awareness; it's about recognizing that our thoughts and feelings are part of a larger story, one that we have the power to rewrite with self-love.

Understanding thoughts

Developing the ability to understand the origins of our thoughts and how to question them is essential. Thoughts arise from the brain's neural network, influenced by past experiences, ingrained beliefs, and current circumstances. Recognizing that thoughts are not fixed truths is important, as it allows us to observe them without getting hooked or becoming aware when a particular thought triggers a cascade of negativity and bad feelings.

The brain's role in shaping thoughts

The brain's neural network is a complex web of interconnected neurones that communicate through electrical and chemical signals. This interconnected system generates the thoughts, emotions, and behaviours we experience. Once a neural pathway is created, it becomes easier for the brain to produce similar thoughts, as it tends to follow the path of least resistance. The more a particular pathway is used, the stronger and more automatic it becomes. For instance, if you frequently engage in self-critical thinking, these neural pathways become more robust. Consequently, when you encounter a triggering situation, your brain is more likely to default to these well-established pathways, making it easier to generate self-critical thoughts. Conversely, cultivating positive thoughts and behaviours strengthens those pathways, making it easier to think positively in the future.

Our thoughts are shaped by the following factors:

- Past experiences: Every experience we have leaves a mark on our neural network. Positive experiences can create pathways that lead to optimistic thoughts, while negative experiences can form pathways that trigger self-critical or fearful thoughts.
- Ingrained beliefs: Over time, repeated thoughts and behaviours solidify into beliefs. These beliefs become deeply embedded in our neural network, influencing our automatic thought

patterns. For example, if you've repeatedly been told that you're not good enough, this belief can become ingrained and automatically influence your thoughts about yourself.

- Current circumstances: Our present environment and current state of mind also impact our thoughts. Stressful situations can activate negative thought patterns, while supportive environments can be more conducive to positive thoughts.

The brain's plasticity, or its ability to change and adapt, means that we can also reshape these pathways. When consciously practising new thought patterns, we can weaken the old, negative pathways and strengthen new, positive ones. This process, known as neuroplasticity, highlights the importance of mindfulness and restructuring how we think and feel and, therefore, is essential in body dysmorphia recovery.

Understanding how thoughts form and the circumstances of their formation can help you to start to observe and question your thoughts more effectively. This can help you detach from negative thinking and develop a more balanced mindset. Observing thoughts without judgement, you create a space between yourself and your thoughts. The key is to recognize that these thoughts are temporary and do not define you. This is an observational practice that helps create a mental distance, allowing you to see thoughts as fleeting mental events rather than fixed truths.

Looping thoughts

Looping thoughts, also known as rumination, are repetitive, often negative, thought patterns that cycle endlessly in the mind. These thoughts can feel like a broken record, playing the same worries, fears, or self-criticisms over and over again. Unlike normal passing thoughts, looping thoughts stick around, drawing your focus back to the same unsettling themes, such as past mistakes, perceived flaws, or future anxieties. These persistent thoughts can feel overwhelming, consuming mental and emotional energy and preventing you from moving forward. For many, looping thoughts create a sense of being stuck in their own mind, unable to break free from the repetitive mental chatter that amplifies distress.

Looping thoughts often arise as a way for the mind to process unresolved emotions or unmet needs. They can be triggered by stress, anxiety, past traumas, or ingrained beliefs about oneself. These thoughts can act like a signal flare, highlighting areas of our emotional landscape that need attention but are often misunderstood or ignored.

At their core, looping thoughts are a feeling wanting to be acknowledged. They represent the mind's attempt to gain control, make sense of something that feels unresolved or threatening, or a form of self-punishment for letting your guard down. However, when we react to these thoughts or identify too closely with them, we unintentionally give them more power, reinforcing the loop and making it more difficult to break free.

Exercise: Observing thoughts

Find a comfortable position, close your eyes, and take a few deep breaths. Imagine you are lying on your back in a peaceful meadow, looking up at the sky. As a thought arises, picture it as a cloud drifting across the sky. Simply observe it without judgement, acknowledging its presence but not engaging with it. Watch the cloud continue its journey until it is out of sight, allowing each thought to come and go. If you find yourself getting caught up in a thought, gently bring your focus back to your breathing. After a few minutes, gradually bring your awareness back to your surroundings, open your eyes, and take a moment to notice how you feel.

Challenging thoughts

Once you can observe your thoughts, the next step is to question their validity. Not all thoughts are true or helpful. When challenging negative thoughts, you can start to change your thinking patterns. Ask yourself:

- Is this thought accurate?
- Is it helpful?
- What evidence supports this thought?
- What evidence contradicts this thought?

This process, known as cognitive restructuring, helps you move away from automatic negative thinking. Cognitive restructuring encourages you to critically evaluate your thoughts and replace them with more balanced and constructive ones. Practise reframing negative thoughts by writing down each self-critical thought and then writing a counter-statement that is supportive and compassionate. For instance, if the thought is, 'I hate my body,' counter it with, 'My body is my home, and I am working on treating it with kindness.'

You are not your thoughts

It's key to understand that you are not your thoughts. Thoughts are transient and do not have to dictate your identity or actions. Learning to observe and question your thoughts can help you to develop a healthier relationship with your inner dialogue and build a foundation for positive change.

The ability to have agency over your thoughts is crucial as we transition into exploring the underlying issues related to body dysmorphia. This new-found skill will guide you towards deeper self-awareness and resilience, ultimately supporting your healing journey and nurturing a more compassionate and supportive self-view.

Exercise: Tracing and challenging negative beliefs

To practise reflexivity and uncover the roots of your negative beliefs, try this comprehensive exercise. It will help you dig deep into the origins of your negative thoughts, understand how past experiences and ingrained beliefs shape your current self-perception, and challenge the validity of these beliefs. Take out your journal and follow along with these steps:

1. Identify a negative belief: Write down a specific negative belief you have about yourself. For example, 'I feel unattractive.'

2. Ask why: Question why you hold this belief. Write down your initial thoughts.
    -   Why do I think my body is unattractive?
    -   Example response: 'Because I don't look like the models I see on social media.'

3. Dig deeper: For each answer, ask why again. Repeat this step several times to dig deeper into the origins of your belief.
    -   Why do I think I need to look like the models on social media to be attractive?
    -   Example response: 'Because I believe that is what society considers beautiful.'

4. Explore the roots: Continue tracing back your answers until you uncover the underlying experiences or ingrained beliefs.
    -   Why does society's definition of beauty impact me so much?
    -   Example response: 'Because I have always been compared to others and told that I don't measure up.'

5. Reflect on the patterns: Reflect on the patterns you've uncovered. Consider how these past experiences have shaped your current beliefs.
    -   Example reflection: 'I realize that my belief that my body is

unattractive stems from constant comparison and societal standards imposed on me from a young age.'

6. **Challenge the belief:** With this new understanding, start challenging the validity of the negative belief.
   - Is this belief accurate?
   - Is it helpful?
   - What evidence do I have that contradicts this belief?
   - Can I find examples of different body types being celebrated?

7. **Reframe the thought:** Based on your evaluation, reframe the negative belief into a more balanced and constructive one.
   - Example: 'I may not look like the models on social media, but my body is unique and valuable. There are many different body types that are beautiful and celebrated.'

When you engage in this exercise regularly, you can start to see how past experiences shape your current thoughts about your body and begin to develop a healthier, more constructive self-image. Over time, this process becomes easier to do in your head, allowing you to quickly identify and challenge negative beliefs as they arise.

Control and perfectionism

Having understood the nature of our thoughts and learnt the importance of present moment awareness, we now turn to the concept of control in the context of body dysmorphia and explore how the desire for control manifests and impacts our self-image.

Control, whether conscious or subconscious, often emerges as a response to the chaos and unpredictability of life. It is a fundamental aspect of human psychology that provides a semblance of stability, but when it becomes excessive, it can distort our perception of ourselves and sustain negative thought patterns. Similarly, perfectionism, a close relative of control, drives the relentless pursuit of flawlessness, often at the expense of mental and emotional well-being.

In this section, we will examine how control and perfectionism shape the experience of body dysmorphia, the protection they falsely offer, and the significant disadvantages they bring. Through understanding these dynamics, we can begin to untangle ourselves from their grip to aid recovery.

The nature of control

For many, the need for control can stem from past experiences. Events like trauma, bullying, discrimination, or emotional neglect might contribute to a heightened desire for control as a way to maintain safety and stability. It acts as a protective mechanism, preventing a person from feeling vulnerable or exposed to further emotional pain. Through maintaining control, individuals believe they can shield themselves from rejection, criticism, or failure. This control often shows up in various ways, such as establishing strict routines, avoiding certain situations, and meticulous planning. Traits like perfectionism, attentiveness to detail, and high conscientiousness frequently reflect this need for control, helping someone feel more secure and organized in their daily lives.

Control in body dysmorphia

Control in body dysmorphia often involves managing, perfecting, or hyper-fixating on physical appearance. Controlling aspects like dieting, building muscle, or excessive grooming is a way of seeking safety, stability, and improved self-worth. This behaviour provides them with temporary relief from insecurities and fears, offering a perceived mastery over their environment. Despite its negative consequences, control creates an illusion of comfort and order, making individuals feel secure and in control in an otherwise unpredictable world.

How control manifests

- Strict dieting: Adhering to rigid dietary rules to maintain or alter body shape.
- Excessive exercising: Engaging in intense workout routines to achieve a perceived ideal body.
- Frequent mirror checking: Constantly scrutinizing one's appearance to ensure it meets set standards.
- Avoidance: Staying away from social situations or activities that might expose perceived flaws.
- Excessive grooming: Spending an inordinate amount of time on personal grooming to meet self-imposed standards of appearance.
- Use of enhancements: Turning to anabolic steroids, diet pills, or cosmetic procedures to achieve an ideal body.
- Relationships: Seeking reassurance or validation from partners and loved ones due to body insecurities or hesitating to engage fully in relationships out of fear of being judged for perceived physical flaws.

Disadvantages of control

While the need for control may provide temporary relief, it has significant drawbacks:

- Increased anxiety: The constant need to control appearance can lead to heightened stress and anxiety.
- Isolation: Avoiding social interactions to maintain control can result in loneliness and social withdrawal.
- Burnout: The relentless pursuit of control is exhausting and can lead to physical and emotional burnout.
- Distorted self-image: Overemphasis on controlling appearance can exacerbate body dysmorphia, making it difficult to see oneself objectively.

Exercise: Letting go of control

1. Identify control areas: List areas where you feel the need to exert control (e.g. diet, lifestyle, exercise, relationships, appearance).

2. Assess impact: Reflect on how these control behaviours impact your life and mental health.

3. Small steps: Choose one area to loosen your control. Here are a few examples to get started:
    –   Diet: If you have strict dietary rules, allow yourself one meal a week where you eat without any restrictions. Pay attention to how this makes you feel.
    –   Exercise: If you adhere to a rigid workout schedule, skip one session or swap it for a leisurely walk.
    –   Lifestyle: If you have a tight daily routine, allow some flexibility by taking spontaneous breaks or doing an unplanned activity.
    –   Relationships: If you find yourself seeking constant validation, try to hold back and trust that your worth is not determined by others' opinions. Allow yourself to be vulnerable with others, sharing your true self without always needing reassurance.

4. Reflect: After a week, journal about how this change has affected your stress levels and self-perception. Consider questions like:
    –   Did you feel less anxious or more stressed? Why?
    –   How did it impact your overall mood and self-view?
    –   Did you notice any new thoughts or feelings about yourself?

The role of perfectionism

Perfectionism plays a significant role in body dysmorphia. It pushes people to seek an unattainable ideal, creating a cycle of constant self-criticism and dissatisfaction. This self-punishing mindset becomes a way to manage future emotional pain, as someone hopes that by being perfect, they can avoid feelings of inadequacy or unworthiness. However, this pursuit often strengthens negative thought patterns and amplifies the inner critic, hindering the healing process.

Perfectionism also acts as a coping mechanism, where the need for control leads to relentless self-assessment. This mindset fuels ongoing dissatisfaction and mental strain, contributing to the worsening of body dysmorphia. In attempting to shield themselves from feelings of inadequacy, they reinforce the very patterns that damage their mental health.

How perfectionism manifests

- Setting unattainable goals: Striving for goals that are unrealistic, leading to persistent dissatisfaction.
- Persistent self-criticism: Continuously focusing on perceived flaws and shortcomings.
- Constant comparison: Regularly comparing oneself to others, often leading to feelings of inferiority.
- Avoidance of new experiences: Fear of failure or not meeting high standards can prevent someone from trying new things, pursuing further learning, or embracing change.

The social media effect

The pressure to appear perfect is amplified by social media, where curated perfection is the norm. This environment naturally oozes unrealistic standards and contributes to the constant comparison trap. Social media can distort self-perception, making you feel inadequate when you don't measure up to the polished/filtered images you see online. Dating and hookup apps also have a role to play by emphasizing physical appearance and creating a competitive atmosphere. Users often feel compelled to present an idealized version of themselves, which can lead to increased self-scrutiny and heightened body dysmorphia symptoms.

Some parts of these platforms can be very toxic, dismissive, and categorical. The use of tribes and hashtags like 'hung' and 'muscle' can potentially cause distress, further heightening feelings of inadequacy and self-doubt. Moreover, algorithms often prioritize and promote idealized content, reinforcing unrealistic standards and continuing the cycle of comparison. The relentless pursuit of perfection on these platforms can create a sense of inadequacy and be a driving force for body dysmorphia, even if the user is unconscious of this at the time.

The role of the gay scene

Parts of the gay scene can be toxic too, significantly driving perfectionism and body dysmorphia. Clubs and parties often feature chiselled, idealized bodies in advertisements, creating a standard far from the diverse LGBTQ+ community. The emphasis on physical appearance, driven by a desire for sexual appeal, allows a culture of comparison. Some environments can make people feel excluded if they do not fit the norm of muscled bodies dancing with shirts off. Equally, in clubs with dark rooms, it's very easy for someone to feel casually dismissed from an interaction, leading to negative thoughts. Additionally, substance use is very common in these spaces, which can be a temptation for someone wanting to feel comfortable in their environment, potentially leading to addiction and other psychological consequences.

The psychological toll

The pursuit of perfection often leads to:

- Increased anxiety and stress: The pressure to be perfect can create significant mental strain.
- Impaired relationships: Perfectionism can create walls, making it difficult to form authentic connections with others.
- Inhibited personal growth: Fear of failure can prevent individuals from learning and growing through new experiences, often resulting in regret and missed opportunities to follow their dreams.

- Decreased self-worth: Constant self-criticism undermines self-esteem and reinforces negative thought patterns.

Overcoming perfectionism

Overcoming perfectionism involves embracing imperfection and cultivating self-compassion. This shift allows individuals to:

- Recognize achievements: Acknowledge and celebrate progress, not just perfection.
- Practise self-compassion: Counter self-critical thoughts with kind and supportive statements.
- Set realistic goals: Focus on attainable and meaningful goals rather than unattainable ideals.
- Accept mistakes: Understand that mistakes are part of the learning process and do not define self-worth.

Exercise: Embracing imperfection

1. Identify a perfect goal: Choose a goal related to your appearance or achievements that embodies perfectionism. Write down why this goal feels important to you and what you hope to achieve by attaining it.

2. Unpick the need for perfection: Reflect on why the need for this achievement feels necessary. Write down the underlying beliefs and fears that drive this need. Consider where these beliefs come from and how they have influenced your self-image. Journaling about these reflections can help you understand and challenge the need for perfection.

3. Set a compassionate goal: Reframe your perfect goal into a more compassionate one and into smaller, realistic, and attainable steps. Instead of aiming for an ideal that is unattainable, set goals that nurture your well-being – for example, focus on incorporating more fruit and vegetables into your meals and reducing sugary beverages initially rather than attempting a very restrictive diet.

4. Reflect with self-compassion and soothing: Keep a journal to track your accomplishments and progress towards your goal. Focus on effort and improvement rather than the perfect outcome. When self-critical thoughts arise about not meeting your perfect goal, counter them with kind and supportive statements.

5. Celebrate small wins: Acknowledge and celebrate small achievements and moments of progress. Recognize that each step forward is valuable and has a cumulative effect on your health and mindset.

Challenging societal standards

True healing involves opening our minds to diverse perspectives. One way to achieve this is by challenging societal norms with the aim of redefining health, beauty, and self-worth in more inclusive and affirming ways. As gay men, the pressure to conform to these narrow ideals can be particularly intense, often resulting in feelings of never measuring up and becoming overwhelmed.

Societal standards often impose unrealistic ideals of beauty and health, leading to feelings of inadequacy and low self-esteem. It's crucial to question these external benchmarks and realize that these ideals are often unrealistic and exclusionary, and shaped by cultural, social, and historical contexts. Recognizing the importance of defining your own standards, which celebrate diversity, is vital for developing a healthier relationship with yourself and your body. Being gay, this means understanding that traditional standards often exclude or misrepresent our experiences and identities. Embracing diverse perspectives not only challenges these harmful norms but also enriches our understanding of what it means to be healthy and beautiful. This inclusive approach promotes a more holistic and caring view of oneself, which is crucial for self-acceptance.

Exercise: Scrubbing societal assumptions

This exercise can help you examine and challenge societal expectations.

1. Create a list: Write down all the societal expectations and standards you feel pressured by (e.g. beauty, success, behaviour).

2. Scrutinize each expectation: For each item, ask yourself:
    - Why do I feel this way?
    - Whose voice is this (society, family, media)?

3. Identify biases: Recognize any biases in these standards and how they affect your self-perception.

4. Challenge the standards: Ask yourself:
    - Is this expectation realistic or fair?
    - Does it align with my values?
    - How can I redefine this standard to be more inclusive?

5. Redefine your standards: Write down new definitions of beauty, success, and self-worth that reflect your values.

6. Reflect regularly: Revisit this exercise periodically to stay aligned with your personal values.

Expanding perspectives: the role of positive psychology

To further enhance this journey of challenging societal norms, incorporating positive psychology practices can be immensely beneficial. Positive psychology focuses on building resilience and nurturing a more optimistic outlook, which can significantly boost self-esteem and improve self-perception. Practical examples of positive psychology might include the following:

- Building resilience through gratitude practices: Regularly practising gratitude helps shift the focus from perceived flaws to positive aspects of our lives. For example, keeping a gratitude journal to note daily positive experiences can reframe your thinking and enhance your overall well-being.
- Promoting hope with achievable goals: Setting small, realistic goals provides a sense of accomplishment and progress. This is important as it creates feelings of hope and increases motivation.
- Leveraging personal strengths: Identifying and using your personal strengths can boost self-esteem and self-worth. Recognizing and celebrating your unique abilities and qualities can counteract negative self-perception and provide a sense of fulfilment and vitality.

Actively questioning societal norms and integrating positive psychology practices, we can create a more inclusive and validating narrative for ourselves and others. This process of broadening our perspectives and embracing diverse viewpoints is key for challenging societal standards and developing a more inclusive understanding of health, beauty, and self-worth. It also prepares us for the next section, which focuses on forgiveness and understanding the ego while learning to diminish its control over us.

Expanding perspectives: mindset matters in healing

Just as societal standards can restrict our perception of health and beauty, labels such as body dysmorphia, anxiety, and depression can confine our sense of self. These labels, often shaped by external influences, can start to dictate our internal narrative if left unchallenged. Labels can be helpful at the start of a healing journey, providing a language that helps individuals make sense of their struggles and playing an important role in offering clarity and validation. They can serve as a lifeline, providing a framework that makes overwhelming feelings more understandable and manageable, especially during times of feeling lost or overwhelmed.

However, as time passes, these labels can begin to define a person, tethering them to a version of themselves that feels stuck, unworthy, or broken. What once served as a helpful tool to understand pain can slowly start to reinforce a narrative of being trapped in the past. The familiarity and validation of these labels can provide comfort during difficult moments, offering a way to categorize experiences and maintain a sense of control when life feels chaotic. Yet they can also prevent deeper engagement with the underlying emotions and root causes of those feelings. For example, attributing everything to anxiety can become an easy fallback, shielding us from confronting deeper issues like unresolved grief, fear of failure, or unmet needs that may be driving the anxiety in the first place.

Letting go of these labels involves compassionately unpicking them and recognizing that they are not the entirety of your identity. This process requires patience and self-kindness, acknowledging that these labels served a purpose but no longer define your journey. Start by gently questioning how these labels impact your daily life – ask yourself if they still serve you or if they are holding you back from embracing a fuller, more dynamic version of yourself. Compassionate self-reflection helps create the space needed to see beyond these labels, allowing you to redefine your narrative with self-compassion and acceptance.

Reflection: Unpicking personal labels

Take a moment to identify the labels or diagnoses that you resonate with, such as body dysmorphia, anxiety, or depression, and reflect on how they impact your self-view. Consider whether these labels still serve you or if they feel limiting. Gently question their role in your life: do they help you understand yourself, or do they keep you attached to past narratives? Imagine how your self-perception might shift if you began to let go of these labels with compassion, seeing your experiences as part of a broader journey rather than a fixed identity.

The power of forgiveness

As part of the gay man's healing journey, forgiveness must be approached with delicacy to truly address the core mental health concerns. Forgiveness is a complex and deeply personal process that involves letting go of resentment, anger, and the desire for revenge against someone who has wronged us but also forgiving ourselves. It's an intentional and voluntary process that can lead to emotional healing and improved mental health.

What happened to you in the past, both good and bad, has shaped you into the person you are today. Your resilience is a testament to this. However, past events can also add emotional weights that hinder mental health and lead to struggles with self-acceptance. These emotional weights may manifest in several ways, such as anxiety, depression, or even our self-perception. As we struggle with thoughts around a particular issue, we may find ourselves overwhelmed, unconsciously leading to control patterns or negative actions/thoughts about our body. This often occurs when there hasn't been closure on a particular issue or if a pervasive sense of injustice lingers.

The benefits of forgiveness are not just emotional; they also extend to mental health. Research has shown that forgiveness is linked to better mental health outcomes, including reduced depression, anxiety, and stress (Griffin *et al.* 2015), as well as to better physical health outcomes such as lower blood pressure (Lawler *et al.* 2003).

However, the journey to forgiveness is not a straightforward one. It often feels like a burn – painful and searing at first – as it forces us to confront our wounds, unresolved emotions, and the ego's instinct to protect us. Staying with this discomfort is a sign that we're engaging with the hurt that needs healing rather than burying it. Although the sting may be intense, it's an essential part of releasing the grip these wounds have on us and allowing ourselves to heal in a way that goes beyond mere thought or rationale.

Practising forgiveness allows us to reclaim our power and free ourselves from the toxic grip of bitterness. This doesn't mean excusing harmful behaviour but rather choosing to let go of its hold on our emotional well-being. When forgiving, we are not condoning the actions that hurt us but rather choosing to move beyond them. This act of letting go is incredibly empowering, lightening our emotional load and creating space for healing and positive experiences.

Forgiveness is a dual-faceted process: it involves both the forgiveness of others who have contributed to our pain and insecurities and self-forgiveness. Self-forgiveness is a cornerstone of healing. It's about acknowledging our imperfections and understanding that our worth isn't diminished by our perceived flaws. This means wholeheartedly forgiving yourself for everything you have put yourself through and acknowledging you were just doing your best with the tools you had at the time. Forgiveness means recognizing your humanity and accepting your mistakes – an essential step in breaking the cycle of self-criticism and negative self-talk that often accompanies body dysmorphia.

This process isn't easy and often needs to become part of a daily practice. We may want to forgive but feel something hasn't shifted within us to fully embody forgiveness. This can lead to shame when we think we should have moved on yet still feel affected. It's important to be patient with yourself here, recognizing that forgiveness is not a one-time event but a journey that requires time and repeated effort.

Different tools and practices can facilitate this journey of forgiveness. Self-reflection, therapy, meditation, psychedelic retreats, breathwork, and mindfulness can all contribute significantly to this process, allowing the expression of pain from past events while simultaneously opening up to love and compassion. For me, these modalities cumulatively provided a sense of clarity and perspective, highlighting the preciousness of the human experience and how grievances that once tormented me seem trivial in the grand scheme of life. Approach these practices with caution and under professional guidance to ensure a safe, legal, and supportive environment.

Forgiveness also involves understanding our role in conflicts and viewing our actions with compassion. This is pivotal in recovering from body dysmorphia. Recognizing that we often act out of pain or fear allows us to forgive ourselves more readily. When we embrace our vulnerabilities and imperfections, we cultivate a kinder relationship with ourselves and others, as further discussed in Chapter 6.

Ultimately, achieving a state of forgiveness is about learning to understand and manage your ego – the voice inside your head that perpetuates self-criticism and negative thought patterns, making forgiveness challenging. When cultivating self-compassion and practising forgiveness regularly, you can begin to dismantle the barriers that hold you back and move towards a more peaceful and fulfilling life. Forgiveness is not only about resolving past hurts but also about creating a more loving and accepting relationship with yourself, treating yourself with kindness, and reducing the ego's control over your thoughts and actions.

Ego games: demoting the inner saboteur

The ego is the part of our psyche that mediates between the conscious mind, the unconscious mind, and reality. It is the sense of 'I' or 'self' that we experience daily. The ego is responsible for our sense of identity, self-worth, and self-esteem. It shapes how we perceive ourselves and the world around us. While the ego can help us navigate social interactions, assert ourselves, and protect us from perceived threats, it can also lead to self-sabotage and negative self-perception when it becomes overactive or unbalanced.

The ego thrives on comparison and validation. It constantly measures our worth against societal standards and the expectations of others. This can lead to feelings of inadequacy, especially when we fail to meet these often unrealistic ideals. The ego's need for validation can drive us to seek approval from external sources rather than finding self-worth from within.

The ego likes to hold on to grudges and be hard on you for making mistakes – all this is a big protection wall in a bid not to be in a similar situation again. This is where it's linked to body dysmorphia: by creating the mindset of never being good enough, it tries to protect you from future pain and anguish – or so it thinks. It amplifies our perceived flaws and fuels a cycle of negative self-talk and self-criticism.

This persistent negative dialogue can distort our self-image and lead to unhealthy behaviours and mental health issues.

I like to describe the ego as a lazy, spoilt child – a voice in your head that you battle with daily. It doesn't like discomfort, including moving out of its comfort zone, which can be applied to trying new things, healing, and feeling pain or facing criticism. The trick is taking the lessons from being able to observe your thoughts and demoting the ego from the boss of you to your assistant manager, so when you feel it's being hard on you for not doing something, learn to appreciate it as not getting its own way and sulking. You can notice the ego by thinking of going to have a cold shower or an early morning gym class – the resistance that you just felt in your mind was your ego. By learning to appreciate this resistance as a tantrum rather than a command, you can begin to diminish its control over you.

Applying this to your healing process involves recognizing when the ego resists change or growth. When you encounter resistance while trying new therapeutic practices, opening up about your struggles or facing painful emotions, acknowledge that this is your ego's discomfort. Viewing these resistances as tantrums, you can push through the discomfort and continue on your healing journey. This approach helps you to embrace the necessary steps for healing rather than being held back by the ego's desire for comfort and familiarity.

Exercise: Understanding your ego

1. Identify the voice:
   - Next time you have a critical thought about your body, pause and pay attention.
   - Write down the exact thought you had.

2. Name your ego:
   - Give this critical voice a playful name, like 'little critic'. This helps you separate the ego from your true self.

3. Dialogue with your ego:
   - Have a written conversation with your ego about this specific body criticism. Ask it why it feels the need to say these things.
   - Respond with understanding but also assert your true values and self-worth. For example: 'Why do you think I need to be thinner? I value my health and strength.'

4. Challenge its claims:
   - For each critical thought, ask if it's really true. Is it based on facts or just feelings?
   - Write down evidence that contradicts these negative thoughts. For example, 'I may not fit the societal ideal, but my body is capable and has brought me joy in many ways.'

5. Appreciate its intentions:
   - Acknowledge that your ego is trying to protect you, even if it's misguided.
   - Thank it for its efforts but explain that you're in charge now. For example: 'Thank you for trying to keep me safe from criticism, but I choose to appreciate my body as it is.'
   - Remember this step and say this affirmation out loud the next time you are stuck in a negative thinking cycle.

The liberation that comes with forgiveness and diminishing the ego's control is transformative. It allows us to move beyond the narrow confines of accepting our thoughts as a given, creating space for a more authentic and compassionate self-perception. This autonomy over our thoughts makes us feel lighter and more self-accepting, especially as we navigate the challenges of body dysmorphia. As we move into the next section, we'll explore how this new-found freedom and self-acceptance enable us to be vulnerable.

Embracing vulnerability

Being vulnerable means allowing ourselves to be seen, imperfections and all. It means being open to experiencing a full range of emotions, including fear, shame, and uncertainty. For gay men, vulnerability can be especially daunting due to societal pressures and discrimination. The walls we build to protect ourselves often become barriers to true connection and healing. They keep others at a distance and hinder our ability to form meaningful relationships. These barriers might be reinforced by past experiences of bullying, rejection, or trauma. Breaking down these walls requires courage, a willingness to face our fears, and trusting in others.

The potential risks of being vulnerable include the possibility of being hurt, misunderstood, or rejected. Admitting to struggles, such as body dysmorphia, can feel like exposing a deeply personal and painful part of oneself. Questions like, 'Will I be taken seriously?' or 'What will they think of me?' may run through your mind, along with the fear of dismissive comments such as, 'Oh, you're not fat' or 'You look great – what are you worried about?' These reactions can feel invalidating and may discourage further openness. However, the rewards of embracing vulnerability far outweigh these risks. Vulnerability leads to authenticity and connection. It allows us to build deeper, more meaningful relationships and to receive the support we need. When we are open about our struggles, we create opportunities for others to relate to us and offer their help and understanding.

Asking for help

Asking for help is a significant step in embracing vulnerability. It requires admitting that we cannot do everything on our own and that we need support. For those dealing with body dysmorphia, acknowledging the issue and seeking assistance can be incredibly challenging. It involves not only recognizing the problem but also trusting others enough to share it with them.

Identifying and accepting body dysmorphia as part of one's experience is a courageous act. It means facing the reality of the situation and being honest with oneself about the need for change. This acceptance is the first step towards healing. Often, we might find ourselves casually joking about our body image issues, which can be a coping mechanism. However, it's important to take these feelings seriously and address them with the gravity they deserve. Acknowledging the true impact that body dysmorphia is having on you and seeking help is vital and one of the first steps in the healing journey.

Sitting with pain and uncertainty

Vulnerability involves accepting that discomfort is part of the journey. It is in these moments of vulnerability that we find our true strength. Confronting discomfort without judgement is crucial in the healing process. Often, we shy away from pain and uncertainty, trying to numb or avoid these feelings. However, sitting with these emotions and acknowledging them without judgement is essential to feeling more at ease and comfortable in our own body, learning to navigate through the core of body dysmorphia, and nurturing a deeper understanding of ourselves.

Our emotions are powerful indicators, each carrying a unique message about our internal state and needs. Anger often reveals where we feel powerless; anxiety highlights areas of imbalance; fear uncovers what is important to us; sadness signifies a need for change or healing; and apathy can signal that we are exhausted and overwhelmed. To truly heal, it is essential to listen to these emotions and understand the messages they are conveying about our needs, guiding us towards the areas of our lives that require attention and care.

Understanding these emotional indicators is vital because it allows us to address the root causes of our distress rather than merely treating the symptoms. Paying attention to what our emotions are telling us helps identify patterns and triggers that contribute to body dysmorphia and other mental health challenges. This self-awareness empowers us to take proactive steps in our healing journey.

Embracing vulnerability is not a sign of weakness but a testament to our courage and willingness to heal. It allows us to move beyond the limitations of our self-imposed walls and into a space where healing and connection are possible, paving the way for a more authentic and fulfilling life. Vulnerability is the gateway to true healing, as it enables us to confront and work through our deepest fears and insecurities with compassion and gentleness, creating a space for growth and more meaningful relationships.

Exercise: Heart-centred vulnerability meditation

This short meditation helps you navigate your vulnerability by focusing on your heart space, encouraging openness and compassion.

1. Sit or lie down in a quiet, comfortable space where you won't be disturbed. Close your eyes and take a few deep breaths, inhaling slowly through your nose and exhaling through your mouth.
2. Place one hand on your heart. Breathe deeply into your heart, imagining your breath flowing directly into your heart.
3. Bring to mind an area in your life where you feel most vulnerable. Allow yourself to acknowledge this vulnerability without judgement. Visualize this vulnerability residing in your heart space.
4. Continue to breathe deeply, directing each inhale into your heart. Feel your heart space expanding with each breath. Ask your heart what it feels about this vulnerability. What words or feelings arise?
5. Silently repeat any compassionate phrases or words that arise from your heart. For example:
   - 'It's okay to feel vulnerable.'
   - 'I am worthy of love and acceptance.'
   - 'I am safe and supported.'
6. Sit with these feelings for a while, breathing into your heart space. Allow yourself to fully experience and embrace the emotions that arise.
7. Slowly bring your awareness back to the present moment. Wiggle your fingers and toes, and when you feel ready, open your eyes.

Take a moment to reflect on how you feel. Notice any changes in your perception of your vulnerability and the words that came from your heart.

The impact of rejection

I think it's vital that we discuss the impact of rejection, as it underpins many of the reasons why a lot of us suffer with body dysmorphia. Put simply, rejection hurts, but it's a part of life, from job interviews, applications, friendships, unexpected betrayals, or even with regards to sex, dating, and relationships. The sting of rejection can vary, often depending on our level of investment, past traumas, or self-confidence. For many, each rejection accumulates, becoming a cumulative unconscious wound that affects us deeply unless we address it.

Think back to your youth. Perhaps you were rejected at a party for not fitting in, made to feel foolish on your first day of school because you were different, or picked last for sports teams due to perceived stereotypes. Maybe you were bullied about your appearance, ridiculed for your clothes, your mannerisms, or the way you carried yourself. These early experiences of rejection can leave deep scars, especially if they relate to aspects of ourselves we cannot change – our sexuality, gender expression, appearance, or other inherent traits. For gay men, such rejections can be particularly damaging, leading to a pervasive sense of not being good enough. The pressure to conform to heteronormative standards often amplifies these feelings, making it harder to accept and love ourselves as we are.

In regard to body dysmorphia, rejection can be especially debilitating. Rejection can come from critical comments or felt through exclusion based on looks. Each instance of rejection reinforces the belief that one's body is inherently flawed, leading to a cascade of negative thoughts. Even if the rejection isn't directly related to looks or the body, those with body dysmorphia can easily find it an opportunity to make controls or restrictions – for example, the infamous breakup diet.

The mindset lessons from this chapter are designed to help you unpick both longstanding and future rejections, particularly by helping you trace back to the core where rejection stings the most. The following steps will also guide you in building resilience and keeping you mindful:

- Acknowledge the hurt: Allow yourself to feel the pain of rejection without dismissing it. It's okay to be upset or hurt – these feelings are valid and part of the healing process. Take some time to reflect with your journal on what happened and why it hurt so much.

- Reflect on the intent: Try to understand whether the rejection was meant to be constructive or if it reflects the other person's issues more than your own. Ask yourself if the rejection was truly about you or more about the other person's insecurities or circumstances. This perspective can help in not internalizing the negative feelings.
- Build self-worth: Focus on your strengths and accomplishments. Remember that your value is not defined by others' opinions. Celebrate your achievements, no matter how small they may seem. Create a list of things you like about yourself and refer to it whenever you feel down.
- Seek support: Connect with loved ones who appreciate you for who you are. Sometimes the unconditional acceptance of a pet can also be a great comfort. Reach out to friends or family members who uplift you and understand your struggles. Sharing your feelings with someone you trust can lighten the emotional load. Additionally, consider discussing these feelings with a therapist, who can provide a safe space for exploring your emotions and offer valuable insights and coping strategies.
- Practise self-soothing: Develop techniques to calm and reassure yourself during times of rejection. Over time, this will help to reduce the intensity of the hurt. This could be anything from taking deep breaths, meditating, engaging in a hobby you love, or even taking a walk in nature. Find what works best for you and make it a regular practice.
- Consider a time when you kindly rejected someone: Reflect on a situation where you had to reject someone kindly and thoughtfully. Remembering this experience can help you understand that rejection is often not about the person being rejected but about circumstances or personal limitations. This can offer a more compassionate perspective on your own experiences of rejection.

Rejection is an unavoidable part of life, but by unpacking the meaning of it and strengthening our resilience, we can lessen its impact on our self-esteem and body image. This can help minimize the pain of future rejection and reduce the influence of past instances on how we view ourselves.

Willingness to change

Overcoming body dysmorphia begins with a genuine desire to improve. Without this foundational drive, progress becomes difficult. The path to changing your mindset is challenging but ultimately worthwhile. This means moving out of your comfort zone, addressing coping mechanisms, understanding why you think the way you do, and beginning a healthier dialogue with yourself. It's essential to understand that wanting to get better involves embracing discomfort, challenging your ego, and facing emotions and aspects of your life that you might have been avoiding.

Sometimes, there is resistance to change because body dysmorphia is all you have ever known. Ironically, it can feel safe, offering a way to control and prevent yourself from going deeper with healing. It's important to be curious about what you would be without body dysmorphia. Would it make you feel free from its constraints and allow a more positive outlook, or does it bring a fear of the unknown? For some, body dysmorphia becomes a significant part of their identity. Without it, there wouldn't be a crutch to lean on during uncomfortable or challenging situations.

Letting go of body dysmorphia involves consciously changing your mindset, allowing yourself to trust in the process, and believing in your potential for change. It means seeing beyond the limitations that body dysmorphia has imposed on you and embracing the person you can become.

Your ingrained beliefs aren't going to change overnight just because I told you that they can. You have to commit to changing them, much like you commit to your progress from training in the gym or learning a new skill. A consistent effort helps in reshaping thought patterns, leading to a more supportive and affirming internal dialogue. Slowly, you will be able to see changes in all areas of your life, not just around your body.

There are still days where I become trapped in negativity surrounding my body. For example, I'm well aware that weighing scales are a trigger for me, as they always used to make me neurotic around diet and training at the gym. Even though I'm able to practise mindfulness and take ownership of my thoughts, weighing myself these days can still be a slippery slope. In these moments, I make a conscious effort now to self-soothe rather than sabotage all my efforts.

Understand that setbacks are a natural part of the healing process. There will be days when negative thoughts resurface or progress feels slow. Now that you are more understanding of your thoughts, you may even get angrier when you find yourself getting hooked by them. Recognize these as temporary challenges rather than permanent failures. Be gentle with yourself and allow yourself to feel your emotions. My advice is to be curious about your setbacks rather than see them as failures; the key is being able to trace back the reasons why you're so hard on yourself and move forward with kindness.

Each day is an opportunity to start anew. Progress requires patience and persistence. When you encounter an off-day, use it as an opportunity to practise resilience and reaffirm your commitment to change. The power of curiosity is important – questioning thoughts, motives, and what you think you know about yourself can lead to significant progress and healing

Changing your mindset will be a continuous process of self-reflection, self-compassion, and embracing vulnerability in the right way. Mindset changes become permanent when they are created within a supportive environment, which is discussed in Chapter 9. Engage in self-compassion practices like mindful breathing, journaling, and speaking kindly to yourself. Remember, it's okay to seek help and lean on your support network and professionals.

As we now move to the other side of understanding mindset, we embark on a journey of unmasking ourselves. This journey to authenticity is paramount in securing a healthy self-view and an adaptable and resilient mindset. Embracing who you truly are and shedding the masks imposed by societal expectations will help you build a life grounded in self-acceptance and genuine self-love.

CHAPTER 6

Unmasking Authenticity

THE FOUNDATIONS OF BODY DYSMORPHIA OFTEN PUSH US to mould our actions and beliefs to conform to societal ideals, sacrificing internal peace in the process. For many, particularly within the gay community, the journey to authenticity – being true to oneself – is filled with obstacles and challenges. Yet, however demanding this path to authenticity may be, it is essential for embracing genuine self-acceptance and is a crucial step in your recovery. Authenticity involves more than being truthful with yourself – it's about unmasking the layers of imposed identities and having the courage to embrace who you truly are.

Authenticity means aligning our outer expressions with our inner truths. It involves celebrating our uniqueness and being truly honest with ourselves about who we are - our desires, aspirations, passions, and values. This journey of authenticity has no fixed endpoint; it's an ongoing evolution of learning about oneself and embracing who we are. Part of being authentic means acknowledging all of our story, including the difficult and challenging parts. Moreover, it requires us to confront and wholly accept the shadows within us, the parts of ourselves that we hide from ourselves and others. Facing these internal truths also involves acknowledging the pain we've experienced from others, as well as the pain we may have caused ourselves and others. Healing from this pain – something we may have been avoiding but which lingers in the background, causing subtle distress – can free us from emotional disconnection, anxiety, or unresolved tension in our lives.

This chapter builds on the previous exploration of mindset, helping to strengthen each of the principles as you anchor yourself in authenticity. The aim is to guide you towards accepting yourself fully – to acknowledge your strengths, embrace your unique qualities, and accept your imperfections. My hope is that the end goal will be a deeper connection with yourself, creating harmony with your inner dialogue and feeling a sense of peace within. Unmasking authenticity will ultimately lead you to lead a more fulfilling and harmonious life, where you can feel comfortable in your own skin.

Embracing authenticity is not a linear journey, and it may involve moments of discomfort, disagreement, and vulnerability – all of which are indicators that you're growing and learning about yourself. When these feelings arise, reflect on them with curiosity, recognizing any resistance as part of the process. As always, take things at your own pace, practising self-compassion and allowing your true self to emerge gradually and naturally.

Authenticity in practice

Authenticity requires radical honesty with yourself and a willingness to let go of the need to conform to external expectations. In practice, this involves acknowledging the gap between who you are and who you feel you need to be and working to close that gap by embracing your values, desires, and emotions.

It's not about rejecting who you are in this moment but rather taking control and intentionally guiding your life in alignment with your authentic self. Often, we disconnect from our true selves when being who we are feels too overwhelming, when our lives become too painful to navigate, or when our experiences force us to confront difficult truths. Reconnecting with your true self means acknowledging these struggles and choosing to lead your life in a way that honours your real identity.

Living authentically can promote inner peace because it allows you to live in harmony with your core beliefs rather than constantly striving to meet the expectations of others. This is particularly significant for gay men, where the conflict between internal truth and external pressures can create emotional distress, contributing to challenges like body dysmorphia. Embracing your authentic self is a vital step in healing from this dissonance. There's also power in vulnerability; allowing yourself to be seen, flaws and all, is one of the bravest things you can do.

For many gay individuals, the path to authenticity is uniquely complex. Pressures from both outside society and within the gay community itself can make self-acceptance difficult. Conforming to heteronormative standards or even to specific expectations within the community can feel overwhelming. Authenticity, in this context, means bravely expressing your identity, desires, and lifestyle choices – despite the potential for judgement or rejection.

It's important to remember that what authenticity looks like for one person may differ for another. Embracing this diversity of experience is part of the journey. Your path is uniquely yours, and learning to honour it without comparison is a strength.

Choosing to be authentic is a revealing and continuous process but often unsettling. Personally, I still find it frightening, wrapped in doubt about whether I'm doing the right thing. The masks I wore to avoid rejection or judgement offered protection but peeling them back required vulnerability. At times, it made others uncomfortable, and there are always triggers and temptations to revert, along with the risk of being misunderstood or not fitting in.

For much of my life, I hid or altered parts of myself to conform – whether by silencing aspects of my identity or adhering to standards imposed by society or even my own community. Embracing authenticity often feels like walking a tightrope of fear. This fear shows up daily: holding back my thoughts, avoiding vulnerability, or withdrawing from social situations. But these moments are part of the challenge on the path to authenticity. Instead of retreating into old patterns, I've learnt to acknowledge the fear and move forward with courage – and, most importantly, self-compassion.

Ultimately, I've accepted that I might not always fit in, and I may still face judgement. But that's okay. Authenticity isn't about pleasing everyone – it's about showing up as my true self, even if that means standing apart. It's a risk worth taking for the freedom and peace of mind it brings. The beauty of authenticity lies in having no façade to uphold. You will resonate with some and unsettle others, but none of this affects the essence of who you truly are.

Authenticity's relevance to body dysmorphia

Authenticity is particularly important in the context of body dysmorphia as it highlights the tension between one's true self and the external image we often feel pressured to uphold. Body dysmorphia thrives on this disconnect between societal ideals and personal truths, pushing individuals to mould their appearance or behaviour to meet external standards. This widening gap between how we appear on the outside and who we truly are on the inside can lead to perfectionism, harsh self-criticism, and a constant fear of disapproval. Authenticity, however, embraces imperfection and values intrinsic worth over the need to conform to unrealistic ideals. It encourages self-acceptance and the celebration of your identity and body. Part of the recovery from body dysmorphia is the journey towards authenticity – discovering what it means for you, independent of external pressures and expectations.

Authenticity as a control mechanism

The inner turmoil of struggling with authenticity can often lead to body dysmorphia being used as a control mechanism. When we feel disconnected from our true selves – unable to express our emotions, identity, or desires – we may turn to controlling our appearance as a way to regain a sense of stability. This behaviour and its related actions become an outlet, offering a temporary sense of control when other aspects of life feel chaotic or beyond our grasp.

For example, someone might focus intensely on achieving a 'perfect' body as a way to compensate for deeper emotional struggles. The effort to mould the body to fit external ideals can become an attempt to control how others perceive them, masking the discomfort of feeling inauthentic or unworthy. Obsessing over appearance can divert attention from unresolved emotional pain, such as fear of rejection, loneliness, or self-doubt. The perfectionism that body dysmorphia often encourages becomes a way to manage these deeper, more painful emotions, even though the relief it offers is only temporary.

Using body dysmorphia as a control mechanism can provide the illusion of security. By obsessively tweaking or criticizing physical features, some may feel as though they are 'fixing' something tangible rather than facing the complexity of their emotional landscape. It's a coping strategy that allows avoidance of more challenging inner work, such as addressing feelings of inadequacy, low self-worth, or the fear of not fitting in. Yet this control is ultimately an illusion, as it never truly resolves the underlying emotional conflict.

For instance, someone who feels deeply uncomfortable in social situations might focus on their appearance as a way to protect themselves. If they can perfect how they look, they believe they can avoid judgement, rejection, or scrutiny. The temporary relief gained from external validation – whether through compliments or the avoidance of negative judgements – soon fades, leaving the individual still feeling disconnected from their authentic self.

This need for control becomes even more powerful when it becomes a collective pursuit. In communities where chasing the 'perfect' body is normalized, it no longer feels like an individual struggle or a coping mechanism but instead feels like a natural part of life. When those around you are also fixated on achieving an ideal, it reinforces the belief that self-worth is tied to appearance. Over time, the behaviours that stem from deeper emotional struggles – restriction, overexercising, and body obsession – become so ingrained in the culture that they no longer feel like survival strategies, just the way things are. This shared pursuit makes body dysmorphia feel valid and necessary, masking the deeper emotional struggles driving it.

Recognizing body dysmorphia as a control mechanism is a key step in breaking free from its grip. It requires a shift in perspective – from viewing appearance as something to be controlled to seeing it as just one small part of your broader identity. When you recognize that control over your body won't solve deeper emotional struggles, you can begin to let go of the need to constantly 'fix' yourself.

Shifting the focus: embracing your strengths

Shifting your focus from perceived flaws to recognizing your unique strengths is a powerful step towards authenticity. Embracing what makes you distinct – both physically and emotionally or intellectually – can help you develop a more compassionate relationship with yourself. Rather than striving for perfection, take pride in the qualities that make you feel strong, proud, and whole.

In moments of self-doubt or when faced with harsh self-criticism, practise kindness towards yourself. Exploring acts of self-acceptance, such as affirmations, self-forgiveness, or gratitude, helps shift your mindset and build a more authentic relationship with yourself, grounded in appreciation rather than judgement.

Creativeness as a path to authenticity

As part of embracing authenticity, we open up space for something deeply personal: creativity. Creativity is one of the most powerful ways to express our authentic selves and an important tool in healing. Whether through art, music, writing, or another form of creative expression, engaging in creative activities helps us explore and express parts of ourselves that may otherwise remain hidden, perhaps due to fear of criticism, a lack of belief in ourselves, or even unawareness brought on by clouded thinking. It's through creativity that we can tap into our inner world, bringing light to thoughts and emotions that may feel too difficult to articulate in words. Creative expression allows us to access deeper layers of our psyche, making the intangible more tangible, and in doing so, it offers relief and insight. Beyond self-expression, creativity also offers a sense of purpose – allowing us to channel our inner experiences into something meaningful and transformative. When we create, our attention shifts away from how we appear or how we imagine others see us. Instead, we are immersed in the process of self-expression, releasing emotions and thoughts that might otherwise remain trapped, offering a sense of freedom that goes beyond the surface.

There are countless forms of creative expression, and the key is finding the outlet that resonates most deeply with you. Whether through the visual arts, writing, movement, or other mediums, creativity provides a safe space to reconnect with your true self. For some, journaling might offer a way to process emotions regularly, while others may find healing in visualizing their feelings through painting, composing music, or designing something meaningful. What matters most is that creativity provides an alternative way to express what might otherwise be difficult to capture in words, offering healing where traditional verbal processing might fall short.

The importance of self-honesty

Honesty with oneself is the cornerstone of authenticity. Without facing the truth about who we are, what we do, and how our behaviours affect us, we remain stuck in cycles that can keep us from embracing our true selves. This section encourages you to reflect deeply on the choices, habits, and coping mechanisms you've adopted, asking whether they genuinely serve your well-being or if they might be holding you back.

Being honest with yourself means recognizing not just your strengths and positive qualities but also the behaviours and patterns that may be detrimental to your physical and mental health. This includes physical behaviours, such as turning to coping mechanisms like drugs, alcohol, or steroids – perhaps as a way to numb emotional pain, fit in, or manage stress. While these behaviours may seem to offer temporary relief, they often deepen the emotional wounds they seek to ease.

On a psychological level, it's essential to reflect on the patterns of thought or behaviour that might be holding you back. These can include self-sabotaging tendencies, like negative self-talk, perfectionism, or avoiding vulnerability out of fear of judgement or rejection. Recognizing both internal and external behaviours helps you understand what truly serves your well-being and what prevents you from living authentically.

Self-honesty requires you to ask difficult questions, such as:

- What behaviours am I engaging in that may be harming me physically, mentally, or emotionally?
- Am I using substances or actions to avoid dealing with deeper issues like self-esteem, rejection, or fear?

This process is crucial for recognizing harmful patterns, such as substance use, unhealthy eating habits, overexercising, or emotional escapism. Through being truthful with yourself, you can uncover the emotional triggers behind these behaviours, paving the way for genuine healing and change.

Exercise: Identifying coping mechanisms and authenticity triggers

Goal: Understand the ways you respond to emotional triggers and situations where you feel pressure to suppress or alter yourself, while exploring healthier and more authentic responses.

1. Track your actions and feelings: Over the course of a week, pay attention whenever you find yourself engaging in behaviours like using alcohol, substances, overeating, overexercising, withdrawing from social interactions, or other coping mechanisms. Also, note when you feel the need to hide or change parts of yourself. What was happening at that moment? Who was involved?

2. Spot the patterns: At the end of the week, review your notes. Are there recurring situations, emotions, or people that trigger these behaviours? Do certain scenarios prompt you to seek comfort, distraction, or to act differently from your true self?

3. Reflect on your emotions and responses: Consider how you felt before, during, and after each behaviour. Were you seeking to escape, fit in, or avoid something deeper? How do your reactions serve or hinder your emotional well-being and authenticity?

4. Challenge your reactions: The next time you encounter one of these triggers, pause and consciously choose a different, healthier response. How does this new way of reacting make you feel? Does it help you feel more aligned with your authentic self?

5. Celebrate small wins: Each day, take a moment to acknowledge something you've done that feels true to you, whether it's a new response to a trigger or an act of self-compassion. This practice is vital because it shifts your brain's focus towards positive reinforcement, helping to rewire neural pathways

for self-compassion and resilience. Celebrating small wins strengthens the brain's reward system, making it easier to continue with positive behaviours and build lasting change over time.

Helpful hints:

- Notice if certain situations or people consistently lead you to engage in particular behaviours. Recognizing these patterns can help you anticipate triggers and prepare healthier responses.

- Be mindful of whether your actions are helping you face challenges or are allowing you to avoid deeper feelings like fear, rejection, or insecurity.

- Pay attention to how these habits impact your relationships, sense of self-worth, and overall happiness. Are they supporting your well-being or holding you back?

Acknowledging the need for support

A key aspect of self-honesty is recognizing when you can't go on alone. Asking for support is not a sign of weakness; in fact, it's one of the most courageous things you can do. Whether you need help addressing addiction, mental health struggles, or simply navigating the complexities of your emotions, reaching out for support is a powerful step towards healing.

There are various options if you decide to seek support:

- GP (Doctor): Your GP can be an important first step in seeking help. They can assess your situation, offer medical advice, and refer you to appropriate mental health services such as therapy or counselling. GPs can also provide support for managing any physical symptoms related to mental health struggles, ensuring that you have a holistic care plan.
- Therapy: Speaking with a mental health professional can provide practical tools for addressing harmful behaviours and replacing them with healthier coping strategies. Therapy also offers a safe space for exploring difficult emotions and developing a stronger sense of self-awareness.
- Support networks: Leaning on trusted friends or family can help you stay accountable and provide emotional support when needed. Additionally, joining support groups for specific issues – whether in person or online – can create a sense of community and shared experience, reminding you that you're not alone in your journey.
- Charities and non-profit organizations: Many charities and non-profits offer resources specifically geared towards mental health, body image issues, and addiction recovery. Some services are listed in the resources at the back of the book. They often have helplines, counselling services, and peer support groups that can guide you towards healthier coping mechanisms and recovery.

Practical steps towards change

Once you've acknowledged the behaviours that aren't serving you well, the next step is to begin making gradual changes. Reflexivity, which we discussed in Chapter 5, plays a vital role here. Regularly reflecting on your actions, thoughts, and feelings helps you to become more aware of the motivations behind your behaviours and start to shift them. Here are a few suggestions to help you move forward:

- Start paying attention to the emotions or thoughts that arise before you engage in harmful habits. Use reflexivity to pause and assess your reactions in the moment; this awareness helps you to understand the underlying reasons behind your actions.
- Begin by making gradual changes towards letting go of destructive habits – for example, you could start by reducing the frequency or intensity of alcohol or substance use. Replace these with healthier alternatives, like physical activity or creative hobbies, which provide a similar emotional outlet. While this process may be challenging, taking small, manageable steps helps to ease the transition and build momentum towards lasting change.

Being honest with yourself isn't easy, as it often involves confronting parts of yourself that have been hidden for a long time. This process can feel uncomfortable, especially when addressing deep-rooted habits or emotions.

Integrating the shadow

As you explore further this process of self-honesty, you'll inevitably come across aspects of yourself that you've kept buried or perhaps never fully acknowledged. These hidden or repressed parts of your identity – what Carl Jung, a Swiss psychiatrist and psychoanalyst, referred to as the 'shadow' – often contain unresolved emotions, fears, or beliefs about yourself. For many, body dysmorphia is not just a response to external societal pressures but also a reflection of the internal conflicts within the shadow.

The shadow represents the parts of ourselves that we might feel ashamed of or want to forget. These could include shame, feelings of inadequacy, fear of rejection, memories of past criticism, or unresolved trauma. These hidden elements often run deeper than simple feelings of inadequacy; they may be the unhealed scars left by deep emotional experiences. Trauma, especially, has a way of reshaping how we see ourselves, embedding itself into the stories we tell about our worth and desirability. These experiences, when left unaddressed, can contribute to ongoing emotional conflict, further deepening the disconnect between our inner selves and outer expressions.

To integrate the shadow is to stop rejecting these parts of ourselves and, instead, bring them into the light of awareness. This process can be uncomfortable, as it involves confronting feelings of shame, fear, and insecurity. However, by facing these hidden aspects, we not only understand their role in perpetuating body dysmorphia but also begin the process of healing from within. The goal isn't to eliminate the shadow but rather to integrate it – meaning to accept that these deeper feelings are a part of who you are. They don't define your worth or dictate how you should view your body.

Here's how you might begin integrating the shadow:

- Unearth hidden emotions: When your focus shifts obsessively to your appearance, ask yourself: what deeper feeling is this really about? Are you trying to cover up a fear of rejection, or is there an old wound of unworthiness resurfacing? These moments of fixation often act as signposts pointing to unresolved emotional pain. If you're already aware of the deeper feeling, approach it with curiosity – what is it trying to tell you?
- Invite vulnerability: Instead of striving for unattainable standards, challenge yourself to be vulnerable. Allow others and, more importantly, yourself to see the parts of you that don't conform to societal expectations. True strength lies in embracing these imperfections and seeing them as aspects of your humanity, not as failures.
- Rewrite your inner narrative: Your shadow feeds on critical self-talk – the voice inside that tells you you're not good enough. Begin rewriting this narrative by speaking to yourself as you would a close friend. When the harsh voice arises, acknowledge it gently – perhaps saying, 'Thank you for trying to protect me, but I'm okay now.' This compassionate response helps to remind you that your worth isn't contingent on appearance or

achievement. Shifting this inner dialogue, you begin to dissolve the power your shadow holds over you.

- Seek comfort in your wholeness: Integration means bringing together all the parts of who you are – both light and shadow, strengths and struggles. It's not about rejecting the shadow but learning to coexist with it. Accept that you are a complex, multifaceted individual and that no single aspect defines you. The more you come to terms with your wholeness, the less control these hidden parts have over you.

Bringing these hidden parts of yourself into consciousness, you begin to realize that the struggle with body dysmorphia is often not solely about appearance. It's rooted in unresolved emotions, past experiences, and suppressed feelings that need acknowledgement and integration. As you embrace the shadow, you can move towards a more authentic, compassionate relationship with yourself – one that honours the entirety of who you are, not just the surface.

Recognizing shadow traits

As you continue to explore your shadow, it's important to acknowledge the traits or behaviours that may emerge from the parts of yourself that you've kept hidden. These shadow traits are often the parts of our personality that we might find uncomfortable or that others may have pointed out to us. For example, you may have been told that you're too needy, annoying, overly sensitive, or demand attention, often in contexts where vulnerability or emotional expression was discouraged or rejected.

These traits might feel frustrating or shameful, but they often arise as a form of self-protection or a reaction to unmet needs. Failing to recognize and own these traits can lead to self-criticism or the belief that you constantly need to 'improve' yourself to fit in or be more acceptable. This mindset can create a cycle of being overly hard on yourself, constantly striving for perfection while pushing down aspects of who you truly are – a breeding ground for body dysmorphia – making it even harder to embrace your authentic self.

When shadow traits go unacknowledged, they can continue to operate unconsciously, driving behaviours that keep you stuck in patterns of dissatisfaction. Owning these traits, however, allows you to see them as signals for deeper emotional work rather than flaws to fix. It's a necessary step towards self-acceptance and inner peace, helping you embrace your complexity rather than rejecting parts of yourself.

Shadow traits aren't inherently bad. They are simply the parts of us that surface when we haven't fully processed or acknowledged certain feelings. Everyone experiences shadow traits, as they are a natural part of being human. For instance, behaviour that may be seen as 'seeking reassurance' could stem from a deep need for validation or connection, perhaps related to past experiences of rejection or criticism. By gently recognizing these traits, you can start to view them not as flaws but as signals guiding you towards understanding your deeper emotional needs. This shift in perspective allows for a more compassionate and honest relationship with yourself, ultimately paving the way for authentic healing and self-acceptance.

Exercise: Engaging with your shadow traits

1. Identify a pattern: Reflect on situations where you feel you've been called 'too much' or 'not enough'. What were the circumstances? How did these traits manifest?

2. Trace the emotion: Try to connect the trait to an underlying emotion. Is it fear, sadness, or perhaps insecurity that brings out these reactions?

3. Practise self-compassion: Remind yourself that these traits are not reflections of your worth. They are simply responses to unmet emotional needs that deserve kindness and attention.

The light shadow

It's important to understand that shadow traits don't only represent the behaviours we dislike or feel ashamed of. There are also positive aspects, often referred to as the 'light shadow'. These are the qualities we might downplay or feel uncomfortable acknowledging because they don't align with the image we've been taught to maintain. For example, you may be told you're 'too kind', 'too creative', or 'too sensitive' – traits that, when embraced, can actually be great strengths. Both your light and darker shadow traits deserve your attention and understanding.

It's also helpful to gently examine the intentions behind your behaviours. Shadow traits may arise when we act out of fear, insecurity, or the need for validation. For instance, when you find yourself being 'too much' or 'too demanding', it might come from a genuine desire for connection, but perhaps delivered in a way that pushes others away. By examining your intentions, you can start to recognise when you're seeking connection or reassurance and whether you're approaching these needs from a place of insecurity or kindness.

When reflecting on your shadow, ask yourself:

- Am I acting out of fear or love? This question helps you explore whether your intentions are rooted in insecurity or in a more positive desire to connect.
- How do I want to be seen? Often, we act in ways that reflect how we want others to perceive us. Be gentle with yourself as you reflect on whether this need for approval is guiding your actions.
- Do I intend to be unkind or malicious? It's important to consider whether your actions are coming from a place of concern, hurt, or defence rather than a genuine desire to cause harm. For instance, if you've been labelled as 'pestering' while expressing concern for someone dealing with addiction, your intention may stem from care and fear for their well-being, not malice. Understanding this distinction can help you soften your approach to both yourself and others, allowing you to act from a place of compassion rather than self-criticism.
- Can I hold space for my light? Acknowledge the parts of you that shine – your creativity, sensitivity, or compassion. These

qualities might feel vulnerable, but they are integral to who you are.

Shadow work isn't about labelling traits as 'good' or 'bad'; it's about understanding the full range of who you are and accepting both the light and dark sides of your personality. When two people's shadow traits meet, it can create a web of complexity, potentially leading to tension or misunderstandings – especially if unprocessed emotions and judgements are involved. Examining your intentions with kindness can help you navigate difficult emotions and interactions with more self-awareness. This not only softens your approach to your own shadow but also helps you understand the shadows of others with more empathy. Ultimately, understanding your shadow is key to peeling back the layers of body dysmorphia and addressing the internal conflicts that shape how you view yourself and your body.

Confronting your pain

As part of shadow work, feeling your own pain is a necessary but difficult step. This process isn't about wallowing in your suffering but rather acknowledging what you've been through. Suppressing or avoiding emotions only keeps them trapped inside, deepening your suffering. When we turn towards our pain, we begin to release its grip on us, making room for healing.

To truly feel and process your pain, start by creating space for your emotions without judgement. Whether you're feeling sadness, shame, fear, or the sting of past hurts from others, give yourself permission to sit with those emotions, letting them exist without the need to change or fix them immediately. So often, we're taught to suppress or ignore our pain, or we simply lack the tools to navigate it. Instead, allow your emotions to flow naturally, understanding that this act of acknowledgement is the first step towards genuine healing. As discomfort arises, recognize that it's a natural part of the process. Rather than distracting yourself from it, practise mindfulness or meditation, staying present with the sensations in your body. Breathing into the tension, you can gradually release it bit by bit. Naming your pain can also be helpful. Whether it's loneliness, fear of rejection, or anger, identifying the emotion allows it to feel less overwhelming, making it easier to manage.

Allowing yourself to fully engage with your pain, you open up space for healing to begin. This process isn't about staying in the pain forever but about understanding and coming to terms with it. The more you acknowledge and work through your pain, the less power it will hold over your thoughts and judgements, helping you move towards a deeper sense of peace.

Confronting the pain caused to others

Just as important as facing your own pain is acknowledging the pain you may have caused others. Often, when we are in the depths of our own struggles – whether with body image or internalized shame – we may unintentionally hurt those around us. This can include withdrawing emotionally, pushing people away, or projecting our own insecurities onto them.

Being honest about the pain you've caused is difficult, but it is also essential for your healing. It allows you to build stronger, more authentic relationships with others and clears the emotional clutter that may be contributing to your struggles with body dysmorphia.

It's natural to feel ashamed or defensive when reflecting on the pain we've caused. That resistance, however, only serves to keep us stuck in old patterns and prevents growth. To start addressing this, allow yourself to sit with the discomfort that arises when you think about moments where your actions or words may have hurt others. Defensiveness often indicates that we're avoiding uncomfortable truths. It can be challenging to admit when we've hurt someone, but owning our actions without making excuses is vital for healing. The act of taking responsibility creates a space for genuine reflection. From here, you can begin to understand the impact of your actions on others and work towards making amends. If you feel an apology is necessary, approach it with authenticity. However, it's important to consider whether offering an apology is appropriate, especially if the person has distanced themselves from you. In these situations, discussing the matter with a therapist can provide clarity. They can help you determine whether reaching out would be helpful or disruptive to both parties' healing.

Overthinking pain: a barrier to healing

Overthinking both the pain you've caused and your own pain can become a way of avoiding healing. You might get stuck in cycles of guilt, self-criticism, or endlessly replaying past mistakes. This can keep you in the same patterns – overanalysing your actions, obsessing over pain, or fearing judgement. Rather than moving forward, you remain frozen in guilt or regret. For me, overthinking past hurts became a form of self-punishment – a way to blame myself for not foreseeing events that caused pain and for letting my guard down. I had to consciously become aware of this pattern and work to break the cycle.

While self-reflection and accountability are crucial, they must be balanced with self-compassion. Whether you're reflecting on your own pain or the pain you've caused others, acknowledge it, but don't let it define you or turn it into a tool for self-punishment. Remember, you're human – imperfect but capable of growth. Healing is about learning and becoming better, not about punishing yourself. Holding on to the past only delays your progress – go a little easier on yourself for once; allow yourself to forgive and release the weight of overthinking.

Avoiding emotional bypassing and self-dismissal

It's common to encounter strategies that temporarily shield us from our emotions. While these coping mechanisms may provide short-term relief, they can also prevent us from fully addressing our pain. Try to notice if any of the following behaviours subtly creep in during your healing process, as they can hinder your ability to fully confront and process your emotions.

- Toxic positivity: This encourages maintaining an overly optimistic outlook, even when it doesn't reflect how you truly feel. While it's important to maintain hope, ignoring or dismissing negative emotions in favour of forced positivity can hinder your progress. Allow yourself the full range of emotions, not just the 'positive' ones. Healing requires honesty, and that includes acknowledging your pain.
- Self-gaslighting: This occurs when you downplay your own

feelings or convince yourself that your emotions aren't valid. It can arise from shame, fear of judgement, or the belief that others have it worse, leading you to minimize your pain and feel it's not 'bad enough' to warrant attention. To avoid this, challenge your inner dialogue – remind yourself that your feelings are real, and they deserve to be felt and processed, even if they're uncomfortable.

- Numbing through routine: Some people may avoid or gloss over their pain by diving back into their usual routines – whether through work, exercise, or keeping busy – without addressing the underlying emotions. While staying active can be helpful, it's important to slow down and create moments of stillness where you can truly sit with your emotions and process what you're going through.

- Spiritual bypassing: This occurs when spiritual beliefs or practices are used to avoid dealing with difficult emotions or unresolved personal issues. While spirituality can be a powerful tool for healing and self-discovery, it can also become a way to sidestep emotional pain. For instance, using meditation, mantras, or affirmations solely to 'rise above' negative feelings without fully addressing the root causes can prevent genuine healing. Some may adopt the belief that 'it's God's will' or 'the universe has a plan' as a way to distance themselves from their pain. While these spiritual explanations can bring comfort, they can also be used to bypass the need to engage with difficult emotions or process trauma.

- Intellectualizing your emotions: Some people avoid feeling their emotions by overanalysing them, treating their emotions as intellectual puzzles to be solved rather than experienced. While reflection is important, turning feelings into purely mental exercises can create distance from the emotional reality and stall genuine healing.

Shifting the focus: moving beyond self-centred pain

When we're in deep pain, it's easy to become consumed by it, making it difficult to move forward. For example, after a painful breakup, we might start to see other people's actions – whether they seem distant or supportive – as being directly connected to our pain. If someone pulls away, we may feel it's because we're unworthy of attention. If they offer support, we might interpret it as pity, reinforcing our sense of suffering. This inward focus can leave us feeling isolated, as if our pain is at the centre of every interaction.

In these moments, we might dwell on negative emotions or seek constant validation from others, hoping they will somehow resolve our inner turmoil. But this can prevent us from addressing the deeper issues at play and delay true healing.

Focusing too much on our pain isn't about vanity – it's a form of self-protection. We may start to view our pain as the central narrative of our lives, believing no one truly understands what we're going through or that we're always justified in our suffering. While this can feel comforting in its familiarity, it can also block our path to healing and growth.

Recognizing these patterns is important because they often create barriers to recovery. Here are a few signs that you might be stuck in self-centred pain:

- Overidentifying with your pain: When suffering becomes a key part of your identity, it can feel safer to stay in that space rather than exploring the possibility of healing. It's a protective mechanism, but it can prevent you from growing and moving forward.
- Needing constant validation: Continuously seeking approval or sympathy from others for your pain may indicate a reliance on suffering as a way to feel in control or maintain a sense of importance.
- Adopting a victim mentality: Viewing yourself as a victim of circumstances or others' actions can make it difficult to take ownership of your healing. While acknowledging the hurt is necessary, remaining in a victim role can keep you from taking steps towards recovery.
- Shifting blame onto others: If you often find yourself blaming others for how you feel, it may be a sign that you're avoiding taking responsibility for your own healing.

Building self-acceptance

Healing requires humility – recognizing that we don't have all the answers and may need guidance from others. It also means being open to different perspectives on your mental health and actively working to acknowledge your shadow, allowing you to move beyond it.

A fundamental reason for exploring authenticity is to embark on a journey of self-acceptance – embracing all the parts of who you are. This means owning your strengths, weaknesses, quirks, and imperfections and knowing that you are worthy of love and respect just as you are. This quest is challenging; I recall being stuck, unable to embrace my shadow for weeks, after recognizing certain traits in myself that I had long avoided. It was difficult to acknowledge the qualities that I often found frustrating in others in myself. I had to work hard to embrace these aspects, not just the easy things to love or the qualities I felt proud of. Over time, I found that accepting my shadow gave me more patience and compassion, both for myself and for others, when I saw similar traits in them.

Self-acceptance is not a one-time achievement but a practice to nurture daily. As life presents new challenges old insecurities may resurface, and societal pressures may tempt you to revert to patterns of self-doubt or perfectionism. During these times, return to the reflections and exercises discussed throughout this book. Regular check-ins with yourself can help you remain aligned with your authentic self and maintain the self-compassion needed to move through life's ups and downs and inevitable setbacks throughout your journey.

Self-acceptance may take time and effort, but each step brings you closer to a more authentic version of yourself. Healing is difficult, and it's important to remember that it's not a solitary path. If at any point you feel overwhelmed by the emotions or memories that come up, it's okay to pause and seek help. Whether it's a trusted friend, therapist, or support group, you don't have to go through this journey alone. Sometimes having someone to talk to can provide much-needed reassurance as you face the more difficult parts of yourself.

Doing this inner work can lead to deeper self-connection and a greater sense of ease in your relationships. As you embrace the parts of yourself you've previously hidden, authenticity begins to heal your relationship with both your body and others, creating more fulfilling bonds and a stronger sense of everyday peace. Remember, this work takes time, and there is no need to rush. If certain sections of this chapter feel particularly intense, allow yourself to step away, reflect, and return when you're ready. Everyone's journey looks different, so take it at your own pace and remember that taking breaks is part of self-compassion.

Exercise: Daily practices for self-acceptance

Self-acceptance is a daily practice that helps you build a healthier, more compassionate relationship with yourself. These simple exercises – affirmations, body gratitude, and self-reflection – will guide you in shifting from self-criticism to self-love. Incorporate them into your routine to nurture a sense of worth and embrace who you are.

- Affirmations: Begin your day with affirmations that remind you of your worth. Simple affirmations can be:
  - 'I accept myself exactly as I am' – a powerful reminder that you are deserving of love and respect, just as you are.
  - 'It's safe to be in my body and embrace all aspects of who I am' – encourages you to feel secure within yourself and your body, accepting every part of your identity without fear or judgement.
  - 'I honour my journey and trust that I am exactly where I need to be' – reminds you to be patient with yourself.
  - 'I am worthy of love, connection, and kindness – just as I am' – a reminder that your worth is inherent and not dependent on external validation or change.

  Tip: You could print these affirmations and place them in visible spots, like your fridge or office desk, to serve as unconscious reminders throughout the day.

- Body gratitude: Shift the focus from appearance to function. Appreciate what your body does for you each day. Thank your body for its strength and resilience rather than fixating on perceived flaws.

- Self-forgiveness: When you catch yourself in self-criticism, pause and practise self-forgiveness. Acknowledge that everyone has imperfections and that mistakes do not diminish your value.

- Compassionate reflection: When a trait you dislike in others triggers you, take a moment to reflect on why. Is it mirroring something you struggle with in yourself? Use this awareness to develop empathy for both yourself and others.

CHAPTER 7

Mindful Movement

EXERCISE IS A COMPLEX SUBJECT, especially when it intersects with body image within the gay community. While working out undeniably supports both physical and mental health, offering a way to de-stress and feel good, it's not always that straightforward. For many, exercise goes beyond just movement and well-being; it's intertwined with our sense of self, validation, and often the pursuit of an 'ideal' body that often feels expected in some gay spaces, where appearance can feel like a currency.

The pressure to achieve a certain look – often a lean, muscular physique – can turn exercise into a source of stress and anxiety rather than something enjoyable. Not everyone enjoys or feels comfortable in the gym, yet many push themselves to fit into that environment, even when it doesn't feel right. For some, the gym can build strength and resilience, but it can also become a stage for comparison, self-criticism, and potentially harmful behaviours like overtraining, extreme dieting, or steroid use. It's a constant balancing act – trying to embrace the genuine benefits of exercise without slipping into a cycle driven by societal pressures or unspoken demands to conform.

For newcomers to exercise, it can be a particularly intimidating experience. Whether it's the gym, a class, sports team, or other space, the unfamiliar surroundings, equipment, and often unspoken expectations can make stepping into these places feel overwhelming. This sense of unease can be even more intense for those living with body dysmorphia, who may struggle even more to find a supportive environment that encourages a healthy relationship with movement.

This chapter explores the multifaceted relationship between exercise and body image. Whether you aim to build muscle, lose weight, or simply move to feel good, it's essential to approach exercise mindfully, respecting what your body needs rather than chasing an external ideal. We will unpack how to navigate this double-edged sword, finding movement that aligns with your desires – whether that's lifting weights, yoga, dancing, or walking – without the pressure to meet a particular standard. The goal is to embrace exercise in a way that nurtures both your body and mind in a fulfilling and authentic manner that honours your individuality, ultimately redefining your relationship with movement.

Navigating my relationship with movement and the gym culture

Before moving to London, my experience with exercise was limited to the local leisure centre gym, where I would navigate the weight benches mostly on my own. Encounters with other men, let alone other gay individuals, were rare. The gym was simply a space to release pent-up anger and frustration, an escape where I could build a tougher exterior. However, once in London, I became increasingly aware of the gym culture, particularly within spaces frequented by gay men. This shift brought a new layer of anxiety, often unconsciously at first. Suddenly, going to the gym wasn't just about working out – it became a social scene. I found myself dressing up for the gym, hyper-aware of my form and routine – and, most daunting of all, was the locker room experience. Baring my body felt like an invitation for judgement, intensifying my insecurities, even if nobody batted an eyelid or cared about my presence.

I also became aware of how the gay scene overlapped with the gym, where I'd see the same social circles together in the clubs as well as in the gym. Some would say hi and have a casual conversation, while others would never so much as look at you, even if you said hello to them because you were used to seeing them at the same hour every day. Naturally, at the time, I thought this was a reflection on me. I assumed it was because I didn't have a six-pack that I was casually dismissed. Now, I understand that it's not my concern why.

Not only was this a factor I took into consideration when I chose to take anabolic steroids, but it also impacted my relationship with exercise. I stopped training for me and was exercising for other people's approval – unbeknownst at the time. Not only did this affect my health, but I lost joy in movement, and I overtrained because there would be severe mental consequences if I missed a training session. Naturally, this led to injuries and poor recovery.

Healing has taught me several key considerations that are vital in my recovery from body dysmorphia, particularly when it comes to movement. These elements include:

- Choosing movement that challenges and suits my body: I focus on finding exercises that are both enjoyable and challenging and tailored to my individual needs. By choosing activities that suit my body, rather than forcing myself into routines that don't feel right or I don't enjoy, I've been able to sustain a healthy and rewarding exercise habit.
- Focusing on the mental benefits of movement: Recognizing that exercise is not just about physical change but also about boosting mood, reducing anxiety, and improving mental clarity has helped shift my perspective from aesthetics to overall well-being.
- Finding a supportive environment: Exercising in spaces where I feel safe and free from judgement has been vital in rebuilding a positive relationship with movement.
- Using exercise as a social outlet: Exercise has become a valuable way to connect with others, offering a healthy alternative to clubs and parties and helping to build meaningful relationships.
- Setting realistic goals and celebrating progress: Focusing on achievable, personalized goals has helped me stay motivated and appreciate my progress without the pressure of unrealistic comparisons. I've learnt to keep my routine flexible, adjusting it based on how I feel, which keeps exercise enjoyable and prevents it from becoming a chore. Celebrating even the smallest achievements, like personal bests, learning new movements, or holding a handstand in yoga, reinforces my confidence and strengthens my positive relationship with exercise.
- Listening to my body's signals and learning to rest: Paying attention to how my body feels during and after exercise has

been vital in recognizing when to push forward or pull back. Embracing the importance of rest and recovery has helped me avoid overtraining and burnout and maintain a balanced approach to fitness.

- Recognizing and navigating toxic fitness culture: Fitness culture can often feel toxic, driven by constant comparisons, unrealistic standards, and an emphasis on aesthetics over well-being. Influencer misinformation, the relentless pressure to do more, and the glorification of extreme behaviours can lead to overtraining, disordered eating, exercise as punishment, and the use of performance-enhancing substances. Being aware of these toxic elements without getting drawn in has helped me refocus on prioritizing my health and enjoying movement in a supportive environment.

Each of these elements has been key in supporting my recovery from body dysmorphia, helping reshape my relationship with exercise – factors we will explore in more detail in the following sections of this chapter.

Choosing the right exercise: discovering the joy of movement

Whether you're new to exercise or workout several times a week, it's important to reflect on why you want to exercise and how you choose to move. Some of you may genuinely enjoy being part of a team, attending classes, or hitting the gym regularly, while others might find it more of a mental chore, feeling pressured to push their body in ways that feel unnatural or to workout in environments that don't suit them – like feeling obliged to go to the gym because it's the norm or feeling self-conscious exercising in front of others yet still pushing themselves to do so.

Exercise is often framed as a tool for achieving a certain look or reaching fitness goals, but its benefits extend far beyond aesthetics. Physically, it improves cardiovascular health, builds strength, and enhances flexibility, contributing to overall fitness and a more active lifestyle. Beyond the physical, regular movement boosts mood, reduces anxiety, and builds confidence, helping you connect with your body in a positive way. For example, research has shown that even low-intensity activities like walking can significantly improve mental health outcomes (Chekroud *et al.* 2018). Similarly, a meta-analysis of 121 studies also found that exercise enhances body perception and self-image, highlighting its impact on how individuals view themselves (Hausenblas and Fallon 2006). The key to experiencing these benefits is finding the type of exercise that feels enjoyable and sustainable, turning movement into a respectful celebration of what your body can do and less about chasing an ideal.

Movement should never feel like a societal obligation or punishment but rather a personal expression. From dance and yoga to strength training and hiking, each form offers unique benefits, catering to different moods and energy levels. Dance is expressive, yoga promotes mindfulness, strength training builds resilience, and hiking connects you with nature. Exploring different types of movement allows you to break free from rigid ideas of what exercise 'should' be and can transform your exercise routine from a chore into a cherished part of your day.

Reflect on whether the body you want and your exercise choices are driven by personal satisfaction or external validation. Pursuing a body that feels strong and authentic shifts exercise from an obligation to a choice that supports your well-being. Ask yourself: what body do you truly want? Is it strong, agile, and capable, or driven by a desire for acceptance? Misalignment between these desires can lead to frustration, overtraining, and a strained relationship with exercise. Focusing on what feels right for you beyond societal ideals empowers you to build a body that supports your life, reflecting inner values rather than external pressures.

Movement is also a powerful tool for mental well-being, offering a therapeutic outlet for managing stress, anxiety, and depression. The mind–body connection highlights that exercise is not just about physical benefits but also nurturing mental health. Additionally, mindful movements like yoga, tai chi, or walking help you tune in to your breath, sensations, and thoughts, grounding you and offering calm and clarity. This practice helps quiet the mind from negative thoughts, promoting a more balanced mental state – important in body dysmorphia recovery.

What if you dislike exercise?

If you find yourself dreading exercise, start small and explore different activities that don't feel like typical workouts. This can include dancing at home, gardening, playing with a pet, or walking in nature. Focus on movement that feels good rather than intense workouts and build up momentum slowly. The goal is to integrate movement into your daily life in ways that feel enjoyable and sustainable, removing the pressure to conform to conventional exercise.

As discussed in Chapter 5, curiosity around your mindset can provide valuable insights into your relationship with movement. Ask yourself what it is about exercise that feels unappealing – is it past negative experiences, societal pressure, a disconnect between your needs and traditional fitness routines, or a lack of motivation due to other factors such as diet, lifestyle, or energy levels?

Reframing your approach to exercise doesn't mean abandoning what has brought you progress; it's about finding a natural rhythm that supports both physical gains and a positive mindset. Instead of rigid routines, embrace movement that feels good, aligns with your needs, and nurtures your well-being.

Making movement accessible

Not everyone has the same access to movement. Chronic illnesses, disabilities, injuries, or energy limitations can all impact on how and how often someone exercises. While mainstream fitness culture often promotes a 'no excuses' mentality, this fails to recognize that movement should be adaptable, not rigid.

If you live with chronic pain, fatigue, or mobility issues, movement might look different for you. It doesn't have to mean intense workouts or a gym setting. Stretching, chair-based exercises, gentle walking, or mindful breathing can all be valuable ways to engage with your body.

What matters most is finding movement that feels good and aligns with your body's needs – whether that means regular activity or prioritizing rest. Movement should support you, not punish you.

Exercise: Redefining your relationship with exercise

Take your journal and let your thoughts flow freely onto the page. This exercise is about exploring your true relationship with movement – without judgement or pressure. Let your pen move as you reflect honestly on your motivations, your routines, and any fears that hold you back. There are no right or wrong answers, just an opportunity to connect with what feels genuine and fulfilling for you. Here are some prompts to guide you.

- What does exercise mean to you? Reflect on how you view exercise. Is it something you enjoy, or does it feel like a chore?

- Identify your motivation: Do you engage in activities to build a better body or for well-being? Write down your primary reasons for exercising.

- Assess your variety: List the types of exercises or movements you currently do. Are they varied, or do you stick to the same routines?

- Explore enjoyable movements: Identify one new form of movement that excites you. How can you incorporate it into your routine?

- Overcoming barriers: What fears or concerns do you have about switching or implementing an activity you love? What holds you back?

Finding a supportive environment

Research underscores the significant impact that exercise environments have on individuals' mental and emotional well-being, especially for those already grappling with body image concerns. For instance, a study published in the *Psychology of Sport and Exercise* found that the atmosphere of fitness centres – particularly those that emphasize appearance and competition – can intensify body dissatisfaction and self-objectification (Prichard and Tiggemann 2008). The study highlights how environments that focus on aesthetics over health can negatively influence motivation and self-perception, particularly among those vulnerable to body image issues.

Choosing the right environment is just as important as finding the right type of exercise. The spaces we engage in can significantly impact our motivation, comfort, and overall experience. A supportive, positive environment encourages a healthier relationship with movement, helping you feel empowered rather than pressured. Whether it's a peaceful park, a dance studio, or even your living room, finding a setting that aligns with your values and needs can make all the difference in sustaining a positive and fulfilling exercise routine.

Is the gym right for you?

Gym culture can be a double-edged sword. On one hand, it offers a structured environment for building strength and resilience. On the other hand, it often emphasizes appearance, competition, and comparison, which can undermine the positive effects of exercise. Whether you are considering joining or are already a member, it's important to reflect on whether the gym or a specific gym truly aligns with your needs and comfort levels. You may enjoy the gym overall, but certain aspects, like mirrors, a focus on physical transformation, a lack of diversity, and the unspoken social hierarchies, can make the environment feel intimidating rather than supportive, impacting your ability to maintain a positive relationship with movement.

Gay-friendly gyms often feel more inclusive but can also have their own triggers, such as potential cruising in showers, lack of privacy, or social cliques that can feel exclusive. Body image pressures within the gay community, fears of judgement, or even microaggressions around gender presentation can also be present. Conversely, heteronormative spaces may feel less socially charged but can still harbour pressures of comparison, performance, and even subtle or overt homophobia.

While triggers like comparison, judgement, or feeling excluded are real, internal fears and perceptions can sometimes amplify discomfort, keeping you from exploring new environments. For example, you might fear judgement from others even when no one is directly criticizing you or feel self-conscious about not fitting a certain image, which can make you hesitant to try new spaces. Recognizing this doesn't mean ignoring your feelings; it means examining why you feel uncomfortable and questioning whether those barriers are external or rooted in personal fears.

Understanding what makes you uncomfortable in your exercise environment helps you identify supportive spaces that align with your needs and values. Choosing environments that naturally promote a positive connection with movement makes exercise feel more empowering and sustainable, helping you feel strong, confident, and motivated to workout.

Tips on choosing spaces that make you feel supported and comfortable

Choosing the right environment can transform your experience with exercise, making it a source of joy rather than stress. Here are some tips on finding a space that supports your physical and mental well-being:

- Look for inclusivity: Seek out gyms or studios that actively promote diversity and inclusivity. This can be seen in diverse staff and memberships or explicit commitments to creating a welcoming space for all.
- Prioritize atmosphere over amenities: While equipment is important, the atmosphere is key. Spaces that feel welcoming, with friendly staff and a mix of body types and abilities, often provide a more encouraging environment than those that focus solely on performance.
- Explore and create your own safe space: If traditional gyms feel intimidating, consider alternative environments like community centres, outdoor fitness classes, or at-home workouts. Engaging in outside activities or virtual classes can offer a

more relaxed, pressure-free way to move. Creating your own safe space, such as setting up a home gym, following online classes, or joining virtual communities, allows you to exercise on your terms, providing the control and comfort you need to stay connected to movement in a positive way.

- Trial and error: Don't be afraid to try different spaces until you find one that feels right. Many gyms and studios offer trial periods, so take advantage of these to assess how the environment makes you feel – not just physically but emotionally too.
- Listen to your intuition: If a space doesn't feel right, trust that feeling. Your comfort and safety should be the priority and vital in the early stages of recovery when change and new environments can feel overwhelming.

Carefully evaluating your workout environment and being mindful of how it impacts you will help you find a space that not only meets your physical needs but also nurtures your mental and emotional well-being. The right environment can make all the difference in sustaining a healthy and positive relationship with movement.

The social aspects of exercise

Engaging in exercise with others can provide significant benefits beyond physical health, particularly for those recovering from body dysmorphia. Group fitness classes, team sports, and fitness communities, whether online or in person, create a sense of belonging and support that positively influences mental well-being. These environments shift the focus away from self-comparison, highlighting shared goals and encouragement, which can reduce feelings of isolation.

Finding a workout partner or joining classes where you are paired up can also provide motivation and support. These small but meaningful interactions, such as being paired in class, help build a supportive atmosphere and allow individuals to feel seen and included. They can take the edge off any fears about an environment, adding accountability and making movement feel more approachable.

For those who are stepping away from environments or activities that were part of their previous routine, like nightlife or other social settings, fitness communities can offer a different space for connection. This shift provides an opportunity to engage in social interactions that feel more aligned with your current goals and well-being, creating a supportive environment that complements your healing journey. An example could be a workout class that includes a social event afterwards, blending fitness with a sense of community in a way that feels positive and uplifting.

Social connections in fitness aren't just about exercise – they're about building networks of support that reinforce your journey towards better mental and physical health.

Setting realistic, health-focused goals

Setting realistic goals rooted in health rather than chasing aesthetics or perfection is key to building a sustainable exercise routine. Health-focused goals should aim for feeling energized, enjoying movement, and supporting overall well-being. This approach reduces the pressure to constantly push limits, which can often lead to overexercising or burnout. Additionally, health-focused goals are less likely to lead to failure or trigger negative thought patterns.

One challenge is balancing ambition with what's actually attainable. It's important to challenge yourself, but those challenges should be rooted in what's realistic for your body and lifestyle. For example, aiming to increase the weight you lift or adding a new type of movement to your routine are achievable goals that focus on progress rather than perfection. Small, consistent improvements that gradually increase intensity or variety create long-term success.

To illustrate the difference between these approaches, consider the following: a perfection goal might involve setting a target to workout seven days a week with the intention of achieving a highly specific, aesthetic result – such as gaining six-pack abs within two months. This type of goal places immense pressure on reaching an idealized image, which can lead to frustration or feelings of failure if progress doesn't meet these rigid expectations.

In contrast, a health-focused goal could be to exercise three to four times a week in ways that make you feel strong and energized, prioritizing improvements in flexibility, strength, and mental clarity. This shifts the emphasis from appearance-driven outcomes to how the body feels during and after movement, creating a balanced approach. With this mindset, you allow yourself to progress at a sustainable pace without harsh self-criticism, making the journey more enjoyable and rewarding.

Tips for setting realistic goals

- Start small and build gradually: Instead of setting an intense goal right away, begin with manageable steps. If you're aiming to run a 5K, start by jogging and gradually increase your distance. The key is to maintain consistency without overwhelming yourself.
- Listen to your body: Health-focused goals should take into account how your body feels. If you're experiencing fatigue or soreness, it's a signal that your body might need more rest or lower intensity exercise.
- Make it enjoyable: Incorporate activities that you genuinely enjoy. If you hate running, swap it out for a dance class, hiking, or swimming. The more you enjoy your exercise, the more likely you are to stick with it.
- Focus on process, not outcomes: Instead of fixating on a particular outcome (such as losing a certain amount of weight), focus on the process – moving more, feeling better, and gradually increasing your fitness. Outcomes will naturally follow when you prioritize consistency and enjoyment.
- Create a learning environment: Challenge yourself to learn new skills such as a yoga pose or a pull-up. This keeps exercise engaging and rewarding, helping you stay motivated.

Through setting health-focused goals, you're less likely to fall into the trap of overtraining, which can compromise not only your physical health but also your mental well-being. When you focus on feeling good, improving your mood, and maintaining energy, exercise becomes a tool for long-term health, not just a means to an aesthetic end.

Tracking your progress
Weighing/measuring yourself

For many, the scale can feel like an unavoidable measure of progress. This number often becomes emotionally charged, as it can feel like all your efforts – and even your self-worth – are tied to that single reading. If the number doesn't reflect what you expect, it can spiral into frustration, leading to feelings that everything you're doing is ineffective. Toxic fitness culture, which thrives on measuring and quantifying every aspect of your body – from calorie intake to bicep circumference and body fat percentages – only fuels this pressure.

However, while the number on the scale may provide some indication of changes, it's often not the best or healthiest measure of success. Weight can fluctuate due to numerous factors unrelated to actual fat loss or muscle gain. Hydration, hormones, stress, and even how well you slept can all influence your weight on any given day. Relying too heavily on these fluctuations can create unnecessary stress and reinforce the false idea that success is defined solely by numbers rather than by how you feel in your body and mind.

Alternative ways to track progress

Instead of focusing on the scale, consider these other, healthier ways to track your fitness journey:

- Body strength and performance: Keep track of how much weight you're lifting, how many push-ups you can do, or how long you can hold a plank. Progress in strength or endurance is a better indicator of overall health.
- Energy levels and mood: Make note of how energized you feel after workouts and throughout the day. Do you feel more confident or less anxious? These mental and emotional shifts are just as important as any physical changes.
- Clothing fit and flexibility: Rather than weighing yourself, pay attention to how your clothes feel on your body and notice improvements in flexibility or mobility. Feeling more comfortable in your body can be a huge sign of progress.
- Visual progress (without the scale): If visual tracking is important to you, consider progress photos or simply recognizing

changes in muscle definition and posture – these can often tell a more complete story than numbers on a scale.

- Sleep and recovery: Good sleep quality and faster recovery times are strong signs that your body is adapting and thriving with your routine.
- Mind–body connection: Are you feeling more in tune with your body? Are you better at listening to its needs? These improvements in awareness are invaluable in creating a sustainable relationship with exercise.

Stepping away from the scale can be freeing, allowing you to shift your focus to more holistic and meaningful wins related to your progress. Rather than being consumed by a fluctuating number, which can be influenced by numerous factors outside your control, you can focus on the broader improvements in your life and well-being.

Balancing health benefits: finding the middle ground

The benefits of exercise can quickly fade when it shifts from something you genuinely enjoy to something you feel obligated to do. It can easily become more about control than enjoyment, with exercise feeling like the only way to manage how you look or maintain a sense of control over your body – especially when self-image feels unstable or negative. For some, working out might become a daily ritual to stave off feelings of inadequacy, offering only temporary relief. The pressure can intensify when a holiday or event approaches, leading to a surge in exercise as they rush to 'prepare' their body in time.

When driven by anxiety or the fear of not doing enough, it's easy to cross the line into overexercising. Pushing yourself too hard without giving your body proper time to recover often backfires. Instead of seeing the results you're aiming for, your body can't repair itself properly, leading to fatigue, injuries, and ultimately burnout.

The need to see constant progress can leave you feeling trapped in a draining cycle where rest feels like failure. But in reality, rest is not a setback – it's a critical part of long-term success. Taking time to recover helps you prevent injury, avoid burnout, and allows your body to rebuild and grow stronger. Embracing rest as part of the process can transform how you relate to movement, making it more sustainable and fulfilling.

Why rest is just as important as movement

Rest days aren't just about giving your muscles a break – they're when your body does the real work of healing and growth. Without proper recovery, the benefits of exercise can plateau, and you might feel stuck in a cycle of fatigue or injury. These are the key reasons why rest is just as important as movement:

- Muscle repair and growth: Exercise causes tiny tears in your muscles. During rest, these muscles repair themselves and grow stronger, leading to progress. Without rest, you risk fatigue and even muscle loss.

- Hormonal balance and stress management: While all exercise temporarily raises cortisol (the body's stress hormone) to help manage physical stress, overexercising can lead to chronically elevated cortisol levels. This can impair the body's ability to regulate weight by increasing fat storage, particularly around the abdomen, and can make it harder to lose weight. This can be especially frustrating when you're focused on body image, as it may feel like your efforts are working against you. Additionally, if your lifestyle is already busy, stressful, or you have a heightened nervous system, your cortisol levels might already be elevated. Adding intense or excessive exercise to an already stressed system can lead to burnout and overwhelm, making rest and recovery essential for both your body and mind.

- Improved performance: Rest allows your body to replenish energy, reduce inflammation, and return stronger. Without recovery, performance diminishes, leaving you feeling weaker and stalling your progress.

Listen to your body, not just your inner critic

It can be difficult to trust your body's signals when you're constantly feeling like you haven't done 'enough'. You might feel the urge to push through fatigue, soreness, sickness, or injury, believing that rest equates to losing progress. However, your body is always communicating with you. Persistent tiredness, irritability, or struggling during workouts are signs that you may be pushing yourself too hard.

As we age, it's especially important to recognize that our bodies may not recover as quickly or handle the same intensity as they once did. Vigorous exercise routines that used to feel manageable may now require more recovery time. You may find you need to adjust expectations and respect the natural changes your body goes through rather than forcing it to keep up with past levels of intensity.

Instead of ignoring these signals, try to listen to them with kindness. Acknowledge the negative thoughts or guilt that might arise when you take a day off, but don't let them control your decision-making. One indicator of recovery is how you feel in the morning – waking up refreshed, rather than drained, can signal that your body is recovering well.

It's natural to feel like missing a day could set you back, but keep reminding yourself that rest is a vital part of progress. If you're struggling with the idea of complete rest, consider active recovery days. Gentle activities like stretching, yoga, or walking can help you stay connected to movement without the intensity of a full workout, allowing your body the time it needs to heal and recharge.

Rest isn't a sign of weakness. It's a necessary part of taking care of your body, allowing it to rebuild, restore, and grow stronger. Without proper recovery, you risk falling into a cycle where no amount of exercise feels enough. Changing your mindset around rest can be freeing. Instead of seeing rest as lost progress, view it as an essential part of your fitness journey. If you allow yourself time to recover, you'll be more consistent, stronger, and better equipped to reach your goals in the long run.

Fuelling your body for recovery

What you eat before and after exercise is crucial to supporting recovery and overall well-being. Your body needs the right fuel to repair and restore itself.

- Protein for muscle repair: After exercise, your muscles need protein to heal. Include protein-rich foods in your meals to support recovery.
- Carbohydrates for energy: Carbs replenish the energy your body uses during exercise. Whole grains, fruit, and vegetables are great sources of healthy carbs.

- Adequate caloric intake: Proper recovery is not just about the type of food you eat but also ensuring you're consuming enough calories overall. If your calorie intake is too low, your body won't have enough energy to repair muscles and restore glycogen levels, which can lead to fatigue, muscle loss, or slow recovery. Inadequate calories can also impair immune function and increase the risk of injury by leaving muscles and tissues undernourished, making them more prone to strains, tears, and slow healing.
- Hydration: Drink water regularly, not just during your workouts. Hydration helps your muscles function and recover properly. For particularly intense or long sessions, consider incorporating electrolytes to replace lost salts and minerals, which are essential for maintaining hydration, muscle function, and preventing cramps.

Don't fall into diet myths – your body needs a balance of nutrients to recover effectively. Skipping meals or restricting food after a workout can leave you feeling exhausted and slow your progress.

Exercise isn't a race or a punishment – it's an opportunity to connect with your body, feel good, and build strength over time. By listening to your body's needs and giving it what it asks for, you'll find a more balanced, fulfilling approach to movement that supports your long-term health and well-being.

Recognizing and resisting toxic fitness culture

Toxic fitness culture is a major trigger for body dysmorphia, as it can warp the healthy benefits of exercise into an obsessive need for control, constant comparison, and chasing unattainable goals. This environment reinforces unrealistic standards, driving individuals to overexert themselves while feeling perpetually inadequate. It turns exercise into a source of anxiety and self-criticism, particularly for those already vulnerable to body image struggles, heightening the very insecurities they're seeking to manage and potentially leading to the use of performance-enhancing substances, like anabolic steroids, to accelerate muscle growth or fat loss.

Fitness as punishment and the 'earn it' mentality

A key feature of toxic fitness culture is the idea that you must *earn* your food, rest, or even the right to feel good about yourself through exercise. This belief turns movement into something punitive rather than something that nourishes your body and mind. Instead of enjoying the benefits of exercise, you might feel obligated to push yourself, fearing that anything less than maximum effort is failure. In this environment, rest is viewed as weakness, and the pressure to constantly push harder can leave you feeling trapped in a cycle of guilt and exhaustion. When you feel like you need to earn your body's worth through excessive exercise, it becomes a source of stress rather than joy.

Obsession with performance metrics and tracking

Fitness apps and social media often encourage us to track every aspect of our progress – calories burnt, steps taken, miles run. While these tools can be helpful for some, they can quickly turn toxic if you become obsessed with the numbers, using them as a measure of self-worth. This fixation on data can rob exercise of its joy, making movement feel like a series of benchmarks to be met rather than something that makes you feel good. Instead of focusing on how movement improves your mental and physical well-being, the metrics start to dictate whether or not you're doing 'enough'. This is especially harmful for those dealing with body dysmorphia, as the constant pressure to hit certain targets can worsen feelings of inadequacy.

Similarly, sleep trackers, while designed to promote better rest, can also heighten anxiety. A poor night's sleep reflected on an app can fuel feelings of failure or worry about what might have caused it. Instead of waking up and assessing how rested you feel, you might find yourself fixated on the numbers and searching for what you did 'wrong'. Over time, this can create a cycle of stress, where tracking meant to improve health inadvertently causes more anxiety and a sense that you're not measuring up in every aspect of your well-being.

The pressure to always do more

Toxic fitness culture constantly pushes the idea that you should always be doing more – lifting heavier, running further, working out more frequently. This never-ending pursuit of improvement can turn fitness into a joyless task, where you're left feeling like you're never progressing fast enough. The emphasis on relentless progress strips away the sense of accomplishment that should come from physical activity, replacing it with feelings of inadequacy or frustration when you don't meet arbitrary standards.

This pressure is compounded by the glorification of the 'no days off' mentality, where rest is seen as weakness and the idea of pushing through exhaustion becomes a badge of honour. In this mindset, your worth feels tied to how much you can endure and how intensely you can train. While this approach might feel motivating in the short term, it often leads to overtraining, injuries, and burnout – both physically and mentally. Without room for balance, the joy of movement disappears, and the focus shifts to constantly striving for more – more intensity, more workouts, more results – at the expense of recovery.

Influencer culture and unrealistic expectations

Social media is full of fitness influencers who project seemingly perfect bodies, flawless routines, and a lifestyle that revolves around exercise. What's often left out of these curated images are the filters, angles, and edits that create a completely unrealistic standard of beauty and fitness.

Constant exposure to idealized bodies on social media can strongly influence the brain's reward system, especially when we post content and receive validation in the form of likes, comments, or positive feedback. When users upload photos or videos and receive social approval, the brain releases dopamine – a neurotransmitter associated with pleasure and satisfaction. This feedback loop encourages users to seek more validation by posting similar content, reinforcing the pursuit of social approval based on appearance. Over time, this can lead to an addictive cycle, where the desire for external validation drives behaviour, often leading to unhealthy comparisons and dissatisfaction with one's own body.

The pressure to achieve these unattainable ideals pushes many people into unhealthy behaviours in an attempt to fit the mould of perfection to be worth acceptance and happiness. Instead of inspiring self-improvement, social media often leads to self-criticism, turning platforms that should encourage connection into places of comparison, where each post reminds us how far we feel from these unrealistic beauty standards.

Diet and 'clean eating' extremism

Toxic fitness culture often pairs extreme exercise with extreme dieting. There's a strong emphasis on 'clean eating', restrictive diets, or labelling foods as 'good' or 'bad'. This fixation on 'perfect' eating can fuel disordered eating patterns, where food becomes something to control rather than something to enjoy. This can lead to unhealthy relationships with food, where eating is no longer about nourishment but about guilt and restriction.

Hyper-masculinity and the 'ideal' body type

In many fitness spaces, particularly in the gay community, there is often an emphasis on hyper-masculinity – lean, muscular physiques that represent an ideal of strength and power. This can create immense pressure to bulk up, use anabolic steroids, or engage in disordered eating in pursuit of this body type.

If you're larger framed, older, or simply different from the image promoted in mainstream fitness, it can feel like you don't belong in the gym, fitness classes, or other wellness spaces. This sense of exclusion can be particularly harmful to someone struggling with body dysmorphia, as it reinforces the idea that you need to change your body to be accepted.

This idealization of a particular look can be damaging to mental health, as it reinforces the notion that your worth is tied to how you look rather than how you feel or what your body can do. The focus shifts from movement as a way to feel good and stay healthy to movement as a means of achieving a specific aesthetic that often feels unattainable.

Anabolic steroids

Anabolic steroids are synthetic versions of the hormone testosterone. They work by increasing muscle mass and strength while reducing body fat. An estimated 2.9–4 million US residents aged 13–50 have tried non-prescribed anabolic steroids, with around 1 million potentially experiencing side effects (Pope *et al.* 2014). In the UK, it is estimated that 1.1 per cent of individuals aged 16–59 reported using anabolic steroids in 2023, a figure reflecting a nine-year high and highlighting the increased prevalence of anabolic steroid use (Office for National Statistics 2023).

The use of anabolic steroids is significant within the gay community, driven by unique social and psychological factors, with studies estimating that between 5 per cent and 13.5 per cent of gay and bisexual men have used anabolic steroids and up to 25 per cent have considered using them (Kutscher *et al.* 2024). The disproportionate use within this demographic can be attributed to several factors. Body image concerns, muscle dysmorphia, internalized homophobia, and social pressures to conform to specific physical ideals all play significant roles. These pressures are intensified by the visibility of muscular physiques in the gay community, often seen as a symbol of attractiveness and social capital.

Prohormones, often marketed as legal alternatives to steroids, have also become popular among those looking to enhance their physique. These substances convert into anabolic hormones once inside the body, mimicking the effects of anabolic steroids. Although perceived as safer, prohormones carry similar risks, including liver toxicity, hormonal imbalances, and adverse mental health effects. Just like anabolic steroids, their use is driven by the desire to quickly build muscle and align with societal body ideals, making them part of the same conversation about the pressures within the gay community.

Social influence and observations

Many people turn to using anabolic steroids due to social influence, similar to how I was introduced to them. They often become an option through conversations in social circles where someone is seen to be 'successfully' using them, implying their use is acceptable or beneficial. Friends or acquaintances using steroids and appearing to achieve desirable results can create a perception that these substances are an option to improve their physique and perhaps silence any negative thoughts they have about their body. The side effects, which are well documented, don't appear to be enough to deter people. They either seem too severe to actually happen or manageable with other pills and potions, giving the impression that one can control the contra-indications of anabolic steroid use. Admitting steroid use often leads to feelings of shame, unless among a group that openly discusses it. This can lead to denial when questioned by others, particularly doctors or medical professionals, especially when testosterone levels and liver and cholesterol markers are abnormal – possible side effects of anabolic steroid use.

The role of ego: checking your motivation

Part of the decision to use steroids lies in understanding your own motivations. Are you driven by a desire for quicker results – bigger muscles, less body fat – without the time and effort required naturally? Often, these shortcuts are rooted in ego rather than genuine self-improvement. It's easy to convince yourself that a shortcut will give you the body you've always wanted, but it's worth asking: are you using steroids to fill an internal gap, one shaped by self-doubt, insecurities, or external pressures? By questioning this, you may discover that your desire to alter your body is more about meeting a perceived social ideal than personal fulfilment – a choice that carries a range of possible side effects along with the potential for cycles of withdrawal and setback. In these moments, I encourage you to revisit Chapter 5 to help cultivate curiosity about the mindset behind your decision.

Effects of anabolic steroids on the brain

Anabolic steroids impact the brain in significant ways, leading to various physiological and psychological changes:

- Dopamine and reward pathway: Anabolic steroids stimulate the release of dopamine, the neurotransmitter associated with pleasure and reward. This heightened dopamine activity can lead to a sense of euphoria, reinforcing the desire to continue using steroids to achieve the same pleasurable effects.
- Altered serotonin levels: Steroid use can also affect serotonin levels, another neurotransmitter that regulates mood, emotion, and sleep. Alterations in serotonin levels can contribute to mood swings, irritability, and aggression – often referred to as 'roid rage'.
- Impact on limbic system: The limbic system, which controls

emotions and memories, can be significantly affected by long-term steroid use. Changes in this area of the brain can lead to increased aggression, anxiety, and depression.

- Reduction in natural hormone production: Prolonged use of anabolic steroids can suppress the natural production of hormones like testosterone. This suppression can lead to hormonal imbalances, causing symptoms such as fatigue, depression, and a decreased sex drive.

- Neuroplasticity changes: Chronic steroid use can alter the brain's structure and function, affecting neuroplasticity – the brain's ability to adapt and reorganize itself. These changes can have long-term implications for cognitive function and emotional regulation (Mhillaj *et al.* 2015).

Understanding how anabolic steroids affect the brain helps explain the potential for addiction. Combined with the desire to maintain an idealized physique in the gay community, this underscores why anabolic steroid addiction is a critical issue. The fear of losing your hard-earned physique makes stopping steroid use after an 8–12-week cycle daunting and can create an undercurrent of anxiety, often manifesting in body dysmorphia symptoms. This psychological dependency is compounded by the physiological effects that steroids have on the brain, such as increased dopamine levels, which reinforce this behaviour. Additionally, the stigma and shame associated with steroid use can lead to secrecy and denial, perpetuating the addiction. For users with a history of rejection and discrimination for being their true selves, it may become even more difficult for them to reach out for support. The result is that many users tend to go on taking anabolic steroids for prolonged periods, perhaps lowering the dose intermittently to manage side effects while attempting to maintain their physique. Despite the perception of an enhanced metabolism, significant effort is still required to gain muscle mass when using anabolic steroids. Proper nutrition and training are essential, as well as limiting other lifestyle activities such as excess partying and using other substances, including smoking and alcohol, which can further increase the risk of severe side effects.

Questioning your thoughts

Steroids can greatly impact your thinking, making it crucial to regularly question your thoughts to avoid becoming fixated on them.
This mental attachment can lead to severe mental health side effects,
including suicidal thoughts and the inability to question why you are
having these thoughts. Without careful self-reflection and mindfulness, one can quickly spiral into a harmful mental state, highlighting
the importance of maintaining a critical perspective on one's mental
processes while using these substances. Chapter 5 covers mindset in
detail, exploring techniques for understanding and questioning your
thoughts better. Consulting a therapist is highly advisable to navigate
these challenges if you are considering taking anabolic steroids.

Steroid use and club drugs

While anabolic steroids are often used to enhance physical appearance, some users also engage in the use of club drugs – such as ecstasy
(MDMA), cocaine, GHB/GBL, ketamine, speed, and crystal meth – as
part of the party scene. For some, the social pressures of the gay community and the desire to maintain a certain body image coincide with
these substances, creating a dangerous combination that affects both
physical and mental health.

In addition to compounded side effects like cardiovascular and
liver issues, the combined use of anabolic steroids and club drugs can
create a cycle of dependency. Users may start using club drugs to escape
the negative feelings associated with steroid use or to enhance their
social experiences in party environments. Over time, these substances
become intertwined, making it difficult for someone to break free from
the dual addictions.

The combined effects of steroids on body image and the euphoric
highs of club drugs can lead individuals to believe that these substances
are essential for feeling attractive, confident, or socially accepted. However, the brain's chemistry becomes dependent on this combination,
and withdrawal from either substance can trigger severe mental health
issues, including depression, anxiety, and suicidal ideation, while the
physical toll continues to escalate.

Stopping steroid use

Coming off steroids also has its challenges. Not only does testosterone drop, leading to lethargy, but your body will inevitably lose some of the muscle mass you have gained. This puts you in a position where you don't feel like training or sticking to a programme, while simultaneously losing muscle. This is known as a crash for the user, and it is a very sensitive time, particularly for those with body dysmorphia. It's vital during this time to acknowledge these changes and be more gentle with yourself. Engaging in supportive activities such as therapy, maintaining a balanced diet, and seeking support from friends or support groups can help manage the physical and emotional toll. Patience and self-compassion are crucial as the body needs time to readjust to its natural hormonal levels. Monitoring your mental health closely and seeking professional help if necessary can also make a significant difference in navigating this challenging period.

For those who have made up their mind about starting anabolic steroids, the allure of the benefits often outweighs the consideration of negative impacts on the body, and it can be difficult to convince them otherwise. The best advice I can give is to seek as much harm reduction advice as possible. This means educating yourself on the side effects, becoming knowledgeable about safer using practices, and ensuring you are undergoing regular blood testing to monitor any markers that could potentially be out of balance due to steroid use. Some resources to guide you are listed at the back of the book.

Side effects of anabolic steroid use
Physical side effects

- Cardiovascular issues: Steroid use can lead to high blood pressure, increased risk of heart attacks, and strokes.
- Liver damage: Anabolic steroids can cause liver damage, including liver cancer. Elevated liver enzymes are a common sign of stress on this vital organ.
- Hormonal imbalance: Steroids disrupt the natural production of hormones, leading to testicular atrophy,

infertility, and gynaecomastia (the development of breast tissue in men).

- Skin problems: Users often experience severe acne and cysts due to increased oil production.
- Musculoskeletal issues: While steroids can increase muscle mass, they can also weaken tendons, increasing the risk of tendon injuries.

Mental and emotional side effects

- Mood swings: Steroid use is linked to significant mood swings, including aggression, irritability, and manic behaviour. This phenomenon is often referred to as 'roid rage'.
- Depression and anxiety: Users can experience severe depression and anxiety, particularly during withdrawal periods, which can lead to suicidal ideation.
- Addiction: The dependency on steroids can be both psychological and physiological.

Long-term health risks

- Increased risk of addiction: Beyond steroids, users often engage in poly-drug use, increasing the risk of addiction to other substances.
- Chronic health conditions: Long-term use of anabolic steroids can lead to chronic conditions such as cardiovascular disease, liver disease, and metabolic disorders.
- Mortality: Studies have shown that long-term steroid users have a higher mortality rate than non-users, primarily due to cardiovascular and liver-related issues.

Moving away from toxicity: reclaiming movement as self-care

Moving away from toxic fitness culture requires recognizing when exercise shifts from a source of joy to one driven by control, comparison, or external validation. The key is to shift your mindset and approach movement as something that nourishes and uplifts you rather than as a punishment for how you look or feel.

Honouring your body's needs – whether it's asking for rest, gentler movement, or simply celebrating what it can do – helps you cultivate a healthier relationship with exercise. This process involves letting go of unrealistic standards and instead embracing a long-term, self-directed relationship with movement – feeling strong, energized, and at peace with your body rather than constantly pushing for more or comparing yourself to others.

Throughout this chapter, we've explored how movement, especially within the gay community, can be a complex and sometimes challenging aspect of self-care and body image. Exercise should not be reduced to a tool for achieving societal ideals or a means of punishment, but rather embraced as a source of empowerment, joy, and satisfaction in how your body moves and feels.

However, maintaining this balance requires ongoing attention. It's easy to slip back into comparison or overexertion, especially when faced with triggers like social media or changes in your progress. Keeping close tabs on your mindset, being self-compassionate, and surrounding yourself with supportive environments are crucial in sustaining this positive approach. Exercise should always reflect your individual journey, where the true reward lies in how movement makes you feel – not in external markers like aesthetics or numbers.

CHAPTER 8

The Silence Within: Our Biggest Healer

ALL OF MY HEALING EXPERIENCES SO FAR have pointed me towards a single, undeniable truth: to truly break free from the shackles of body dysmorphia and its far-reaching effects, I must learn to embrace stillness. This is more than silencing the constant noise, distractions, and relentless demands of everyday life – it requires having the courage to sit with myself and confront the loudest internal noise. The real challenge lies in facing the discomfort, the fears, and the emotions that fuel the inner critic, giving it space rather than avoiding it. Stillness isn't passive; it's an active and deliberate choice, a potent tool to unlock the healing that has always been within. In the quiet, I finally heard the truth that has been there all along: I am enough.

Stillness involves more than turning off external distractions. It asks us to face the deeper internal barriers we've built – the ones that protect ourselves from confronting our emotions. Burying ourselves in work, endlessly scrolling on our phones, comfort eating, or turning to substances are just some of the ways we may avoid this confrontation. These distractions shield us from the deeper pain, fears, and insecurities, and in doing so, they feed the inner critic.

Creating a safe space for stillness

Stillness requires vulnerability, and it can be overwhelming to sit with emotions we've long avoided. This is why creating a safe space is so important – both externally and internally. Feeling safe allows us to explore our thoughts and emotions without fear of judgement or being overwhelmed.

- External safety: Start by creating a physical space where you feel comfortable and undisturbed. This could be a quiet corner in your home, a favourite chair, or even a spot in nature. Surround yourself with things that make you feel grounded, like a soft blanket, gentle lighting, or calming scents. This external safety helps set the stage for the deeper, internal work of self-enquiry.
- Internal safety: Equally important is cultivating a sense of emotional safety. This means being compassionate and patient with yourself as you sit with discomfort. It's essential to give yourself permission to simply feel without rushing to fix or judge what arises. Internal safety also means choosing moments of stillness when you're not rushing about, stressed with work, or feeling overwhelmed by the demands of daily life. In these calmer moments, you are more equipped to hold space for your emotions and engage with them honestly.

Developing a better relationship with yourself and learning to love the body you inhabit doesn't happen overnight. This is not a sudden shift in perspective, nor is it about adopting a new mindset on demand. Rather, it is a gradual process that begins with learning to listen more deeply – to the thoughts, feelings, and discomfort we have silenced for so long. This process is both beautiful and necessary. In those quiet moments, the distorted beliefs that have shaped our inner world begin to loosen, revealing the truths we've long avoided.

Sitting in silence can be daunting. When you consciously choose to face what you've spent years pushing away, the comparisons, negative thoughts, and judgements may initially feel louder, especially when there's no external distraction to mute them. This resistance is natural; stillness brings vulnerability, and vulnerability can feel threatening when we've spent so long building protective walls. Feelings of impatience – the urge for quick results or the discomfort of unresolved emotions – can also arise. However, stillness teaches patience, reminding us that healing is gradual. The ego often uses discomfort or restlessness as distractions to avoid vulnerability, but facing these emotions offers the greatest potential for healing. In this chapter, I hope to guide you towards seeing stillness not as something to fear but as a space for calm and self-enquiry as you unpack the layers of your inner world.

Stillness as a mind-body reconnection

Stillness is often misunderstood as simply the absence of movement, but in the context of healing, it means intentionally pausing and being fully present with yourself – reconnecting with your body and mind. This creates the space to process your thoughts and emotions in a way that encourages self-awareness and introspection.

For many gay individuals, especially those with trauma or a strained relationship with their body, life often becomes rooted in hyper-vigilance and anxiety. These responses serve as fuel, keeping us alert but disconnected from our bodies. Over time, we start to see our bodies as objects to criticize or fix rather than recognizing them as integral to our lived experience. Stillness offers the opportunity to rebuild that broken connection. When pausing and turning inward, we shift away from the harsh, critical gaze and begin to experience our bodies from within, as they are – worthy of care and compassion.

Reconnecting with the body through stillness also challenges the distorted beliefs that feed body dysmorphia. As we reconnect, we stop viewing our bodies solely through external standards and instead begin to experience them as a vital part of our existence, deserving of love and care. This shift allows us to challenge the negative body image narratives and to begin seeing our bodies as essential to our well-being rather than something to perfect.

This process goes beyond simply taking a break from the noise of life. It invites us to recognize and challenge the harmful stories we've internalized – the distorted narratives about how we should look or who we should be. In stillness, we can examine these stories and gradually rewrite them based on our true selves, not the conditioned beliefs we've carried for so long.

Stillness as an act of defiance

In a world that constantly bombards us with messages about beauty and achievement, choosing stillness is a radical act of self-acceptance.

We're taught that our value is measured by how we look or how much we achieve. To intentionally pause and embrace stillness – to step away from that cycle – is a bold declaration of self-worth. When we reject the pressure to constantly improve or conform, we reclaim our autonomy. Stillness gives us a way to step outside of societal pressures and reclaim our bodies and our identities for ourselves, on our own terms, free from the judgements and expectations imposed by others.

Overcoming barriers to stillness

Stillness is not easy. For many, even the idea of pausing briefly feels overwhelming. The moment we stop, the thoughts we've been avoiding rush in, and the anxieties we've been suppressing come to the surface – especially when those thoughts about appearance dominate. But this discomfort is often a signal that you are on the verge of something important. Resistance is part of the process, often masking deeper truths we need to confront. Understanding this resistance for what it truly is helps ease the fear and leads us closer to deeper healing.

Stillness isn't about doing nothing. It's an active engagement with yourself, a practice of tuning in and listening to what's really going on beneath the surface. If you find the idea of stillness daunting, start small. You don't need hours of meditation or extended silence. Begin with just a few minutes each day. Gradually, stillness will shift from discomfort to refuge, a space where you can reconnect and, ultimately, heal. In this section, we will explore ways in which you can incorporate stillness as part of your healing journey.

How to sit with your feelings

1. Acknowledge the emotion: Start by noticing that something is there. Pause and ask yourself, 'What am I actually feeling right now?' It might be anxiety, anger, sadness, or something else entirely.
2. Name the feeling: Give the emotion a name. Say it out loud – for example, 'I feel anxious' or 'I'm angry right now.'

Naming the feeling can help you better understand and connect with it.

3. Bring curiosity to the experience: Ask yourself, 'Where do I feel this in my body?' Is there tension in your chest, a knot in your stomach, or tightness in your jaw? Notice any physical sensations that come with the emotion.

4. Allow the feeling to be there: Rather than trying to push the feeling away, create space for it. Acknowledge that it's okay to feel this way and that the emotion doesn't need to be fixed immediately.

5. Witness the emotion: Let yourself observe the emotion. If the feeling wants to move – like crying or shaking – allow it. Sometimes simply sitting with the feeling can be enough for it to start releasing.

6. Let go of the need to change it: It's okay for the emotion to be there. You don't need to solve it or make it disappear. Just be with it and trust that it will pass in its own time.

Meditation as a tool for reconnection

Meditation offers a structured way to find sanctuary from the noise of the world and the constant chatter in our minds. In meditation, we create a safe space where self-acceptance can take root. It's a retreat from external pressures and expectations, allowing us to focus on our inner relationship with ourselves.

Meditation is accessible to everyone and doesn't require any special equipment or complicated techniques. Here's a simple approach to get started:

1. Find a quiet space: Choose a space where you won't be disturbed. It could be a room in your house, a quiet corner, or even outside in nature.

2. Sit comfortably: You can sit cross-legged on the floor, in a chair with your feet on the ground, or in any position that

feels natural and relaxed for you. The key is to keep your spine straight with your shoulders relaxed.

3. Close your eyes: Gently close your eyes or soften your gaze by focusing on a point in front of you. This helps minimize visual distractions.

4. Focus on your breath: Begin by focusing on your breath. Notice the sensation of the air entering and leaving your nostrils or feel the rise and fall of your chest and belly. Your breath will serve as an anchor to bring you back to the present moment.

5. Observe without judgement: As you breathe, thoughts and emotions will naturally arise. Instead of trying to suppress them, simply observe them without judgement. Imagine your thoughts as clouds drifting by in the sky. Acknowledge them, then return your focus to your breath.

6. Start small: If you're new to meditation, start with just 5–10 minutes a day. Over time, you can gradually increase the duration as you become more comfortable with the practice.

The purpose of meditation isn't to stop thinking entirely but to create space between yourself and your thoughts. It gets easier with practice, but it's not something to master. Think of it like a workout for your brain – it takes time and consistent effort to train your mind to focus and find calm amidst the noise. Just as with physical exercise, the benefits of meditation build gradually, helping you become more present and compassionate with yourself over time.

Other types of meditation for healing

Meditation comes in many forms, each offering a unique way to reconnect with yourself. Depending on where you are in your journey, certain practices may resonate more deeply than others. Whether you're seeking to reduce anxiety, build self-compassion, or reframe how you relate to your body, exploring different types of meditation can help you discover what works best for you.

- Mindfulness meditation: Focuses on paying attention to the present moment without judgement. Mindfulness helps reduce anxiety by grounding you in the present and observing thoughts without becoming consumed by them. See Chapter 5 for more about mindfulness.

- Guided meditations: Guided meditation can be a valuable option for those who find it challenging to meditate in silence, as it provides structure and direction. It can be particularly helpful to explore guided meditations that focus on body positivity.
- Loving-kindness (metta) meditation: This practice involves cultivating feelings of love and compassion, starting with yourself and then extending those feelings to others. It helps develop a mindset of kindness and empathy, replacing judgement with warmth and care. Loving-kindness meditation encourages you to open your heart and approach both yourself and others with greater understanding.
- Compassionate mirror meditation: If looking in the mirror triggers negative body thoughts, use this exercise to shift your focus. Stand in front of the mirror and, instead of focusing on perceived flaws, look into your eyes with kindness. Repeat affirmations like, 'I am enough as I am.' This practice can transform how you see yourself over time.
- Body scan meditation: Close your eyes and settle into a comfortable lying position. Gently guide your attention through each part of your body, from the top of your head to the tips of your toes. As you move through each area, notice any tension or discomfort, observing without judgement. For areas that feel particularly tight or tense, focus on your breath and imagine breathing into that space, inviting it to relax with each exhale.

You can easily find guided meditations and visualizations on popular platforms like your preferred music service, YouTube, apps, or even podcasts.

Breathwork as a tool for grounding

Breathwork offers a unique way to ground yourself and reconnect with your body. Through controlled breathing techniques like conscious connected breathing – where each breath flows smoothly into the next – you move from observing your body to fully inhabiting it. Unlike meditation, where it's easy to become distracted by the 'monkey mind' or the restless and often scattered thoughts that pull your attention away, breathwork can make it easier to stay present by giving you a clear focus on your breath. This makes it especially helpful when you need something more tangible to keep you centred in the moment.

Breathwork can seamlessly become part of your daily routine, either as a standalone practice or alongside meditation. Its simplicity and accessibility make it a reliable tool for cultivating presence and balance. Breathwork doesn't require a formal setting – it can be practised at home or as part of your meditation routine. However, working with a trained facilitator can deepen the experience, helping you explore breath healing more safely and effectively. Over time, breathwork can become a core practice in your healing journey.

Stillness in everyday life

Stillness doesn't have to be confined to formal meditation practices. There are many ways to invite moments of quiet into your daily life that help reconnect your body and mind.

- Mindful routines: Engage fully in simple daily routines, such as a skincare ritual or shower, without distractions like music or your phone. Focus on the sensations and the care you're giving your body. These small, mindful acts can help you reconnect with your body in a nurturing way.
- Technology breaks: Choose moments where you intentionally disconnect – for example, leave your phone behind during short walks or limit use an hour before bed.
- Breathing exercises: Set aside a few minutes each day to focus on your breath. Notice how your body feels as you inhale and exhale, allowing yourself to become fully present. One helpful method is box breathing, where you inhale for a count of four, hold the breath for four, exhale for four, and pause for four before repeating.
- Mindful eating: Instead of rushing through meals or multitasking while eating, take the time to fully experience your food. Focus on the texture, flavour, and smell of each bite. Mindful

eating can help you stay present and build a more appreciative connection with your body's needs.

- Quiet morning moments: Begin your day with a moment of stillness. Whether it's sitting with your morning coffee in silence or spending a few minutes stretching or journaling, creating a calm space before your day starts can set the tone for more mindfulness throughout the day.

- Nature walks: Take a walk in nature without your phone or distractions. Pay attention to the sights, sounds, and smells around you. This practice not only invites stillness but also helps you reconnect with the world beyond daily stressors.

- Gratitude practice: End your day by writing down three things you're grateful for. This simple practice shifts your focus from what might be wrong or stressful to what is positive in your life. It's a gentle way to wind down and cultivate stillness before sleep.

The transformative power of solitude

Solitude is often misunderstood and wrongly equated with loneliness. In the context of healing, however, solitude is an intentional space for self-reflection. It allows us to turn inward, examine our emotions, and process thoughts we might not be fully conscious of or would otherwise avoid in our busy lives.

Solitude vs. isolation

There's an important distinction between solitude and isolation. Isolation often arises from a desire to avoid difficult emotions, which can lead to deeper loneliness and disconnection. Solitude, on the other hand, is a conscious decision to create space for self-exploration and reflection. Instead of running from our emotions, we meet them directly, giving ourselves the chance for genuine introspection.

For those who fear being alone, solitude can feel daunting. Our culture often encourages constant activity and distraction, leaving little time for self-connection. Yet solitude isn't about withdrawing from the world but rather making room to reconnect with who we truly are.

Although solitude may seem uncomfortable at first, particularly for those used to external distractions, it holds the potential for significant healing. Without the constant noise of societal pressures or the influence of others, we can reconnect with parts of ourselves that are often overlooked or ignored. Solitude offers a chance to see beyond appearance, allowing us to engage with our values, strengths, and desires – the aspects that shape our inner world.

In solitude, we gain clarity about who we are, free from noise. These quiet moments allow us to meet a more authentic version of ourselves, liberated from external judgements. For gay men, especially, solitude offers much-needed freedom – to exist on our own terms, without the weight of societal expectations or the need to conform to external ideals.

What solitude looks like

Solitude doesn't always equate to physical isolation or complete silence. It's creating intentional, quiet moments where you can focus inward, free from distractions. Solitude could involve a peaceful walk in nature, quiet reflection in a cosy corner, or unplugging from technology for a few hours. These moments aren't always about withdrawing from the world entirely but about reclaiming space for yourself to reconnect, process emotions, and deepen your self-awareness.

Strategies for integrating stillness and solitude into daily life

Bringing solitude and stillness into your everyday life doesn't require withdrawing for long periods or undergoing drastic changes. Even small, intentional moments of quiet can help you reconnect with yourself. Here are a few ways to create space for solitude:

- Personal rituals: Establishing personal rituals can serve as a consistent way to incorporate solitude and stillness. Morning meditation or evening journaling can offer structure to your day, creating time for reflection.
- Micro-moments of silence: If carving out large chunks of time seems impossible, micro-moments of silence can be equally effective. These are brief pauses during your day – while commuting, doing housework, or simply sitting quietly – where

you reconnect with your thoughts and feelings. These small breaks provide opportunities to slow down and return to the present moment.

- Solitude as part of your routine: Scheduling longer periods of solitude into your routine can provide more profound moments of introspection. Solo walks, spending time at a quiet café, or simply stepping away from your devices for an afternoon create intentional space to reflect and process without distractions.
- Long-term solitude practices: Consider integrating regular, longer periods of solitude, such as weekend digital detoxes or retreat-style breaks. These extended moments give the chance to go deeper into your inner world, creating an environment for insight and sustained calm.

Exercise: Exploring your solitude

Take a moment to explore what solitude means to you. Solitude is deeply personal, and there's no single way it should look or feel. This exercise will help you reflect on the type of solitude that resonates most with you and how to incorporate it into your life.

1. Find a quiet space: Sit in a comfortable, quiet place where you won't be disturbed. Close your eyes and take a few deep breaths, allowing your body and mind to settle.

2. Reflect on your past experiences with solitude: Think about moments in your life when you've felt at peace while being alone. Were you in nature, immersed in a creative activity, or simply resting in a quiet room? How did those moments make you feel? Write down or mentally note the specific feelings or thoughts that came up.

3. Identify what feels nourishing: Consider the types of activities that help you feel grounded and connected to yourself. Do you find peace in silence, or does gentle movement, like yoga or walking, help you settle into stillness? What role do activities like journaling, gardening, or reading play in your solitude?

4. Experiment with different forms of solitude: Over the next week, experiment with different types of solitude – try spending time in nature, unplugging from technology, or engaging in a quiet hobby. Pay attention to how each experience affects your mood, thoughts, and sense of self. Which form of solitude feels the most restorative?

5. Journal your findings: After each experience, jot down how you felt, what worked, and what didn't. Did you feel more connected to yourself after certain activities? Use this as a guide to create a personal solitude routine that feels meaningful to you.

Sobriety: clearing the noise

Sobriety and silence are powerful allies on the path to healing. Both invite us to strip away the distractions we often rely on to shield ourselves from confronting uncomfortable truths. While not everyone with body dysmorphia has an unhealthy relationship with substances, sobriety – like silence – is a tool that removes the noise that clouds our minds. Whether that noise comes from alcohol, drugs, or any other form of compulsive behaviour, the effect is the same: it numbs us from facing the deeper truths we might not want to see. Some may turn to these behaviours as a temporary escape from emotional discomfort or stress, but the more we rely on them, the more disconnected we become from ourselves.

For me, sobriety didn't come easily or all at once. The thought of giving up alcohol lingered in my mind long before I made the decision to stop. I never considered myself someone who needed to be sober, nor did I fully acknowledge the impact alcohol had on me. Looking back, though, it became clear that alcohol had been a crutch – a way to get through stressful situations and feel more at ease. I rarely entered social situations without it, relying on alcohol to ease my nerves and numb emotions I wasn't ready to confront. At the time, I didn't see it as a problem, but eventually, I realized that rather than helping, alcohol was preventing me from addressing the real issues beneath the surface.

The decision to go sober was one of the most humbling parts of my journey. Not only did I have to explain to others why I was quitting and admit that I couldn't control alcohol, but I also had to confront this truth within myself. It forced me to adopt a complete lifestyle change, one that required not just external adjustments but a deep internal reckoning. Yet, despite the challenges, it has been worth it. Sobriety has given me the clarity to finally tune in to my emotions and the strength to sit with discomfort rather than numbing or avoiding it. I've learnt to face what I used to run from, and in doing so, I've found a deeper sense of peace and resilience.

Sobriety doesn't have to be an immediate, all-or-nothing decision. It's essential to approach it with curiosity rather than pressure. For those who do use substances as a coping mechanism, we can gently explore our relationship with them, examining why we turn to them and what role they play in our lives. Giving up alcohol or drugs can be a significant shift, but it doesn't have to feel overwhelming or become your entire identity.

Sobriety, like silence, offers a way back to ourselves. It clears away the haze and distortion created by substances or unhealthy habits. When we remove these external crutches, we create the space for genuine reflection, and it's in this clarity that we can begin to enhance the healing journey. Sobriety isn't just about abstaining from substances; it's about choosing to be fully present with ourselves, no matter how uncomfortable that may feel at first. This presence, combined with the silence we cultivate, becomes a powerful foundation for transformation.

Practical steps for embracing sobriety
Reflect on your relationship with substances
Start by exploring your connection to substances with curiosity rather than pressure. Notice when and why you tend to drink or use substances – whether it's to unwind, cope with stress, or enhance social situations. For some, this reflection might reveal a problematic relationship with substances, while for others, it may simply highlight areas where more mindful choices could be beneficial. Pay attention to how these behaviours make you feel afterwards and what role they play in your life. Instead of focusing on the idea of complete sobriety, simply observe your habits. Ask yourself, without judgement or pressure, what leaving these behaviours behind might mean for you.

Set small, achievable targets
Rather than focusing on long-term sobriety right away, start with small, manageable goals. For example, commit to staying sober for a week, then gradually extend it to a month. These short-term goals provide a sense of progress and accomplishment without the pressure of a lifetime commitment from the outset.

Set boundaries with kindness
If certain social settings or individuals trigger your desire to drink or use, it's important to create supportive boundaries. Approach conversations with friends or family by focusing on your own journey. For example, saying, 'I'm choosing to focus on my well-being right now, so I'm avoiding alcohol', opens a respectful dialogue. You don't need to

isolate yourself or avoid social gatherings altogether, but having clear boundaries can help protect your sobriety.

Suggest alternative social activities

Instead of avoiding social situations altogether, suggest alternative sober-friendly activities. Invite friends for coffee, a walk, or activities that don't revolve around alcohol or substances. Many people will be open to trying something new, and it helps create a space where you can connect more deeply without the pressure of substances.

Ease into non-alcoholic environments

Trying non-alcoholic environments for the first time can be daunting, but it offers a chance to explore socializing in a more mindful way. Begin by seeking out sober-friendly events or spaces, such as brunches, alcohol-free bars, or wellness-focused activities. Start with small shifts – like opting for a movie night over a party – and gradually expand your comfort in these settings.

Plan for triggering situations

If you anticipate feeling pressure or discomfort in certain environments, prepare in advance. You could bring a non-alcoholic beverage with you or let your close friends know you're choosing not to drink so they can support you. Having a strategy in place can make these situations feel more manageable and help you stay grounded in your goals.

Explore sober communities

Connecting with others who share similar goals can provide valuable support. Look for sober communities or social groups, whether online or in person, that host alcohol-free events or discussions. These groups can be a great source of encouragement, offering both practical advice and a sense of belonging during your journey.

Practise self-compassion

Above all, be gentle with yourself. Sobriety is a process, and it's okay to take it one step at a time. If you find yourself struggling or slipping up, remember that healing isn't linear. Setbacks are a normal part of any healing process. If you do fall back into old habits, remind yourself that it doesn't erase your progress. Instead of focusing on the setback, reflect on what triggered it and how you can prepare for similar situations in the future. Every stumble offers insight into your triggers and provides an opportunity to strengthen your coping strategies. Treat each experience as a learning opportunity, and remind yourself that this journey is about building a healthier relationship with yourself, free from substances.

Seek support

Navigating sobriety can feel challenging, and you don't have to do it alone. Reach out to supportive friends, family members, or communities that align with your goals. Whether it's a close friend who respects your decision or a professional support group, having a network that understands and validates your journey can be incredibly grounding. There's no need to isolate yourself in this process; sharing your experiences and receiving encouragement from others can be an essential part of the healing process. You can find additional guidance on support networks and communities in the resources section at the back of this book.

Once you've experienced the clarity and calm sobriety brings, it becomes easier to stay motivated. However, staying grounded in the 'why' behind your decision to embrace sobriety – whether it's for your mental well-being, physical health, or emotional clarity – will help carry you through the more challenging moments. Remember, sobriety isn't just about avoiding substances; it's about nurturing a deeper connection with yourself, your goals, and your well-being. Focusing on the reasons you chose this path and the benefits you've gained helps you to reinforce your commitment to the healing process.

Silence as a tool for long-term healing

Silence, stillness, and solitude are not just temporary tools for relief; they offer lifelong support. These practices create space for reflection, self-awareness, and connection with your authentic self. Over time, silence becomes a refuge from the external noise, providing a calm environment to process emotions and find clarity.

As you become more comfortable with stillness, it serves as a reliable ally in times of stress or uncertainty. Silence allows for clear introspection, helping you stay grounded and in touch with your true self long after the initial healing stages. It's more than a break from the world – it's a place where you can truly listen to yourself.

Every step you take towards self-acceptance is progress worth celebrating. Silence and stillness aren't just for facing difficulties – they also provide a space to acknowledge your victories, no matter how small. Each time you sit in stillness and engage with your body from a place of compassion, you move forward. Setbacks will happen, but what matters is that you continue showing up, embracing silence, and allowing space for your true self to emerge.

Silence as a lifelong practice

Healing is ongoing, but silence, stillness, and solitude offer continual grounding. These practices are always available, offering a sanctuary when you need a break from the demands of life. Silence becomes a trusted tool for finding inner peace and clarity without the pressures of external distractions.

Whether through meditation, breathwork, or simply pausing in a quiet moment, silence is there whenever you need it. It becomes a companion that supports you in navigating life's ups and downs, providing calm and insight as you continue your journey towards healing.

Exercise: Meeting your higher self

In this reflection, I encourage you to take time to reconnect with your inner voice – the part of you that knows your worth, that understands your struggles, and that holds the wisdom to guide you on your path. This practice of stillness allows you to hear these messages more clearly, without the distractions of external pressures or self-judgement. It's an opportunity to meet your higher self – the wisest, most compassionate version of you who has already walked this healing journey.

Find a quiet space where you won't be disturbed. Sit comfortably, close your eyes, and take a few deep breaths. Begin to imagine yourself standing at the entrance of a beautiful, serene garden. This garden is a special place, created just for you. It's a place where you feel completely safe, loved, and at peace.

The air is soft, and the sun gently warms your skin. As you step into the garden, notice the vibrant colours of the flowers, the lush greenery, and the gentle sounds of nature surrounding you. This is a sacred space where you are free from judgement, comparison, and the burdens of the outside world. Here, you are fully accepted, just as you are.

As you walk deeper into the garden, you see a bench placed under a large, wise tree. This is where you will meet your higher self. Your higher self is the version of you who has already healed from the wounds of body dysmorphia – the version of you who knows the truth of your worth and loves you unconditionally. They are waiting for you here.

When you reach the bench, take a seat, feeling the presence of your higher self beside you, and greet them. Notice their warmth, their calm, and the love they radiate towards you.

Your higher self turns towards you with a gentle smile and invites you to ask any questions that are in your heart. What would you like to know? You may ask your higher self about your healing journey, your relationship with your body, or anything else you've been struggling with.

Now, listen carefully as your higher self speaks. Their words are filled with love, wisdom, and truth. They remind you that you are enough, just as you are, and that you are worthy of love and acceptance regardless of your appearance. They may offer guidance or simply sit with you in compassionate silence. Whatever you hear, trust that these words come from a place of deep knowing.

Take your time to receive the messages they have for you. When you feel complete, thank your higher self for their wisdom and love.

Before you leave the garden, take one final look around. Feel the peace, the acceptance, and the deep sense of connection to yourself. When you are ready, begin to walk back towards the entrance of the garden, carrying with you the love and wisdom your higher self has shared. As you exit the garden, know that this place is always within you, a space you can visit any time you need to reconnect with your true self.

When you are ready, gently open your eyes and return to the present moment. Take a few deep breaths, allowing the peace of this experience to remain with you.

CHAPTER 9

Creating a Supportive Environment

I F YOU NOTICED THE DEDICATION AT THE BEGINNING OF THIS BOOK, you will understand how important I believe the right environment is for healing. This means surrounding yourself with people – whether personal, intimate, or professional – who are genuinely supportive of your well-being. The relationships in your life play a vital role in your healing journey. They can either help rebuild your self-esteem, providing encouragement and understanding, or, sometimes unintentionally, reinforce negative feelings, leaving you feeling misunderstood or unsupported.

Navigating relationships can be difficult, especially when there is a lack of understanding or awareness about body dysmorphia. Well-meaning people might offer advice or reassurance without fully grasping the true emotional impact it has on your emotions and self-esteem. Their responses, though intended to help, can sometimes miss the mark. Comments like 'you look fine' or 'you're overthinking it' may seem supportive on the surface but can unintentionally dismiss the deeper emotional struggles you're facing. This can leave you feeling misunderstood or even invalidated, deepening your insecurities rather than providing the comfort you need. The gap between their intentions and your reality can make it hard to communicate your feelings openly, leaving you more isolated in your experience.

On the other hand, someone who is a bit too honest may unintentionally cause harm as well. A casual remark like 'you've gained a bit of weight' or an offhand comment about an aspect of your appearance can send you into a spiral, reinforcing the very insecurities you're struggling to manage. Instead of feeling supported, such comments can magnify the self-criticism you already face, making it even harder to navigate your thoughts and feelings.

Being in the wrong environment can be just as harmful, if not more. Healing is not only about vulnerability but about feeling truly at ease and safe in your relationships. In the spaces where you feel secure and valued, you're not constantly questioning your worth or assessing your safety. However, when you're in environments where certain pressures, appearance-related expectations, or unhealthy behaviours are normalized, it can cloud your judgement and make it harder to focus on healing. These settings can undermine your sense of self and significantly slow your progress.

This chapter explores how building a support system can shape your healing journey. While relationships alone can't solve the problem, the right connections can provide strength, understanding, and perspective. These networks aren't just a safety net but an active part of your emotional recovery.

Loneliness

Loneliness often starts long before recovery, and it can make the journey even harder. When it comes to body dysmorphia, the isolation can be particularly intense. It's not just the physical solitude that many imagine when they think of loneliness; it's the internal disconnection from those around you, even when you aren't physically alone. It can almost feel like being back in the closet, carrying a secret weight that no one truly understands. You might feel like no one gets the inner workings of your mind or the depth of what you're going through. This kind of isolation can persist into recovery, making the healing process deeply private and almost unbearable, even if you know you are on the right path.

A distinct pattern of loneliness has most likely been present for many of us, but as you confront your struggles, the veil lifts, and it can intensify as you begin to share your vulnerabilities more openly. The risk of vulnerability feels heavy. When you share the depths of your insecurities, there's always the fear that people might not understand, have pity, or worse, dismiss them entirely. This can lead to feeling even more isolated, trapped in your own head, where your struggles remain unseen and unheard.

Another layer of loneliness comes from the fear of being misunderstood or judged. When you're constantly at odds with your own reflection, the idea of opening up to others feels risky. You think, 'What if they don't get it?' or 'What if they think less of me?' or worse, 'What will they think of the real authentic me?' These fears create a barrier to reaching out for help and forming new connections. Over time, this self-imposed isolation can become as painful as the body dysmorphia itself.

One of the hardest aspects of healing is craving deeper connections while realizing not everyone is capable of offering them. Surface-level relationships are no longer enough; you need people who can meet you where you are and who won't shy away from the uncomfortable truths and imperfections of your journey. Yet this craving for meaningful connection also makes you vulnerable to rejection. Not everyone will understand the changes you're going through, and some may even be threatened by it. Healing, after all, often means growth – and growth can make those around you uncomfortable. As you begin to change, some people might not like it; they may have found you easier to tolerate when you didn't set boundaries, blended in with the crowd, and were easier to control.

In some cases, their discomfort may stem from their own struggles, whether with body dysmorphia or other mental health challenges. Your healing journey can act like a mirror, reflecting back their unresolved issues, which can heighten their resistance to your growth. As a result, you may find yourself moving away from environments and relationships that no longer serve you, only to feel the sting of isolation as you haven't yet rebuilt your social network. This is especially true if your healing involves sobriety or stepping away from old habits.

In your journey, you may feel stranded – caught between who you were and who you are becoming – without the comfort of familiarity or the security of new, supportive relationships. This is where hyper-vigilance can kick in: even in social settings, you might never fully relax, always scanning for cues or signs that you aren't safe or accepted. This constant guard can make loneliness even more pronounced, as it feels like you're never truly able to be yourself around others.

You may have developed the ability, or be in the midst of trying, to stop comparing yourself to others' bodies, but there may still remain comparisons about how others live their lives and social situations, especially the filtered angle you see on social media. This can result in more feelings of withdrawal – feeling that nobody shares the same level of doubt or shame as you. It's a vicious cycle: the more isolated you feel, the more negative self-talk takes over, making it harder to reach out and form the connections you need.

Loneliness can also drive you towards unhealthy connections. In the absence of genuine support, you might cling to relationships that are destructive simply because they're familiar. The desire for love and acceptance is so strong that we sometimes settle for any connection, even one that reinforces our insecurities. The comfort of a toxic relationship can seem preferable to the uncertainty of being alone, even though it only deepens the harm.

The problem with loneliness is that the more we retreat, the stronger it grows, convincing us that isolation is our only option. Yet healing begins when you recognize that you deserve real, meaningful connections – relationships that don't demand you shrink or compromise who you are. Yes, being vulnerable is risky, and not everyone will get it, but stepping outside of isolation is necessary for recovery. It's a hurdle you have to pass, embracing the authentic and evolving you.

You don't have to face body dysmorphia or its accompanying loneliness on your own. Healing is hard, but it's not meant to be done in silence. The point of writing this book is to try to put some words to what you may be feeling and perhaps give you a head start on what future you may experience, so you can feel prepared and know that it's all part of the journey. Loneliness was a raw and necessary part of my healing – to learn how to nurture healthy relationships and build a supportive network where I could feel safe and be vulnerable for once in my life.

The sections that follow will hopefully serve as a guide, offering practical suggestions to help you overcome the obstacles of loneliness and isolation on your healing journey. While loneliness may feel overwhelming at times, building a network of allies – people who truly understand, support, and encourage your growth – can help you move forward.

Cultivating a positive healing environment

Human beings are social creatures, and the importance of connection is intrinsic to our biology. Good relationships help protect both your brain and your body, reducing stress, improving mental health, and even supporting your immune system. A famous study, the Harvard Study of Adult Development (www.adultdevelopmentstudy.org), which followed participants for over 75 years, found that those with strong, positive relationships were happier, healthier, and lived longer. The study concluded that 'loneliness kills' – and that meaningful connections are as important to our health as avoiding smoking or drinking.

In body dysmorphia, the psychological benefits of connection can't be overstated. Meaningful relationships provide emotional support, a sense of belonging, and a buffer against the harmful effects of chronic stress and self-criticism. These relationships remind you that you are more than your body, offering a space where you can feel seen and understood beyond physical appearance.

Micro-connections

While deep, meaningful connections are essential, not all interactions need to be significant to have a positive impact. For many, the pressure to build deep relationships can feel overwhelming, especially during periods of emotional strain. However, the benefits of connection can still be felt through micro-connections – those small, seemingly fleeting interactions we have throughout the day. Research has found that brief social interactions, even with strangers, can increase feelings of happiness and belonging (Sandstrom and Dunn 2014). These micro-connections, like a quick chat with a barista or a friendly exchange with a colleague, are simple yet powerful ways to remind ourselves that we are part of a larger social network.

Micro-connections can help break the cycle of isolation, something many of us experienced more acutely during the COVID-19 pandemic lockdowns. While these interactions may not lead to deep relationships, they provide a sense of community and can lift your mood in small but meaningful ways. The key is to remain open to these moments, allowing yourself to engage with others even when deeper connections are not immediately available.

Overcoming the fear of reaching out

Building a support network can feel daunting, especially if you are quite introverted or if body dysmorphia has led you to retreat inward. The fear of reaching out – whether due to concerns about rejection, being misunderstood, burdening someone, or the vulnerability it requires – can make seeking help seem an emotional burden. It's important to acknowledge that these feelings are valid. Many people struggling with body image issues worry that others won't fully grasp their experiences or might downplay their struggles. Additionally, the pressure to appear invincible – to keep up a façade of strength even when struggling internally – can be exhausting and add to the fear of opening up. However, overcoming this hesitation is an integral part of healing. Starting small – by engaging in micro-connections or joining supportive online communities – can help ease the fear of deeper, more vulnerable interactions.

Building your support network

Finding true allies is about surrounding yourself with people who genuinely understand, encourage, and hold space for you. These aren't just the friends, family members, or partners who compliment you – they're the ones who see beyond the surface and who connect with your emotional well-being. It's the people who make you feel seen, not because of how you look but because of who you are. They validate your experiences and encourage your growth, and in doing so, they become a vital part of your recovery.

Take a moment to reflect on your relationships. Are there people in your life who offer empathy and truly listen without judgement? Do they make you feel supported for who you are rather than how you appear? These are your allies – the ones who remind you of your worth and believe in you. While some may not fully understand body dysmorphia, the fact that they're willing to listen and stand by you makes them invaluable.

True allies aren't just there to offer comfort; sometimes they provide tough love as well. These are the people who care enough to have honest conversations with you, even when the truth is hard to hear or when they offer you a perspective you may not wish to take on. They hold you accountable – not in a way that criticizes or diminishes your feelings, but in a way that challenges you to keep growing. They're the ones who remind you of your goals when you start to lose sight of them, and they help you stay on track with kindness and compassion. Accountability is an essential part of healing, and those who genuinely care about your progress won't be afraid to offer honesty in a way that supports rather than hurts you.

And yet, part of healing may mean letting go of certain environments or relationships that no longer serve you. That can be incredibly isolating at first. But it's also an opportunity to create space for new connections, for people who truly understand your journey. Trust plays a huge role in this – trust that there are good, kind people who will support your growth and, most importantly, trust in yourself that you're deserving of these relationships. Building this kind of trust takes time, but it lays the foundation for meaningful connections – ones that don't ask you to shrink or conform to someone else's expectations.

If your current circle doesn't offer the understanding you need, consider exploring online or offline communities that resonate with you. Sometimes it's easier to find people who've walked similar paths in spaces dedicated to healing, like support groups or online forums. Whether it's connecting with people in LGBTQ+ spaces or body positivity communities, there's comfort in knowing you're not alone. These communities can offer a place to share stories, find empathy, and build relationships that reaffirm your worth.

As you create this healing environment – through the people you surround yourself with and the spaces you engage in – you'll likely start to notice subtle but powerful changes. Your self-esteem grows, stress starts to lift, and a sense of belonging takes root. It doesn't mean forcing these connections but instead allowing them to naturally unfold as you move towards spaces that truly support you.

Setting and maintaining boundaries

Boundaries are essential for protecting your mental health in all types of relationships – whether with friends, family, partners, or even acquaintances. They help you define what feels comfortable and safe, allowing you to protect your emotional and physical well-being.

Establishing clear boundaries leads to healthier, more respectful relationships because you set expectations that ensure your needs are valued and understood.

Without boundaries, it's easy to lose yourself in the expectations or needs of others, which can lead to emotional burnout, self-neglect, and a constant feeling of being overwhelmed. People-pleasing tendencies can play a major role here, as you might find yourself prioritizing others' needs above your own to avoid conflict or disappointment. When you don't clearly communicate your limits, you risk overextending yourself to please others, often at the expense of your own well-being. Over time, this can result in feelings of resentment, emotional fatigue, and a sense of betraying yourself. Sometimes this sense of self-betrayal may not be immediate – it can surface later, when a particular event triggers unresolved emotions. These feelings can weigh heavily, and without boundaries, the emotional toll only deepens.

Communicating boundaries in intimate relationships

Intimate relationships can be especially tricky when it comes to boundaries, as issues surrounding body image and physical appearance often feel more intense. In these relationships, boundaries are not only necessary for your emotional safety but also for building trust and mutual respect. It's not always easy to express insecurities about your body, but you have the right to communicate your needs and vulnerabilities openly with your partner.

Being upfront about how certain comments or behaviours make you feel is essential. For example, if remarks about your appearance trigger feelings of insecurity, sharing this with your partner is key to avoiding unintended harm. Standing up for yourself might feel vulnerable, but it's essential for creating a relationship where both you and your partner can feel truly understood and respected. It's not about confrontation but about setting the tone for kindness and support within the relationship.

Respecting both your own and others' boundaries

Setting boundaries isn't just about protecting yourself – it also means respecting the boundaries of others. Learning to accept when someone says no can be difficult, particularly if your hyper-vigilance led you to predict a yes or if you've grown accustomed to pushing your own limits. However, a healthy relationship thrives on mutual respect, where both people feel comfortable expressing their needs without fear of judgement or rejection.

At times, friends or loved ones may express concern about your well-being, especially if they notice behaviours that worry them. Their concern may come from a place of love, and sometimes tough conversations or even interventions can be valuable. However, when their advice is shaped by what they would do in your position, rather than what you actually need, it can add a lot of pressure. What felt right for them may not be what's right for you, and true support means holding space for your journey rather than assuming one solution fits all. The best allies listen, offer guidance, and respect your autonomy, offering support when you are ready.

In some friendships, especially when emotions run high, it can feel easier to cut ties when tension arises or boundaries are crossed. However, hearing no or experiencing discomfort doesn't have to signal the end of a relationship. Disagreements or uncomfortable conversations are natural and can provide opportunities for growth if handled with respect and understanding. Rather than weakening a bond, boundaries can actually strengthen relationships by creating an environment where both parties feel empowered, valued, and more deeply connected.

Saying no to triggering situations

In addition to setting boundaries with others, it's necessary to set them with yourself. This means learning to recognize when to say no to situations that you know will be triggering or harmful to your mental health. Often, these are moments where your body is signalling no but your mind feels like it *should* be saying yes – whether out of guilt, obligation, fear of missing out, or the pressure to fit in. For example, it could be agreeing to attend a social event when you're emotionally drained or continuing a conversation that feels uncomfortable, simply because you don't want to create tension by leaving or disagreeing.

Listening to your body and your emotional responses is key – if something doesn't feel right, it probably isn't. There's no shame in stepping away from situations or environments that compromise your well-being. Boundaries are about honouring your needs, even if those around you don't fully understand or agree with them. Ultimately, setting these personal limits is an act of self-respect, ensuring that you prioritize your mental health above the pressure to conform.

Leaving toxic relationships

One of the most difficult aspects of healing is recognizing when certain relationships – whether friendships or romantic – are no longer serving your well-being. It's not just about distancing yourself from people who don't support your recovery but acknowledging when their presence in your life actively hinders it. Toxic relationships can intensify feelings of insecurity, self-doubt, and negative self-image, making it harder to see your own worth and progress in healing.

Letting go can hurt, but staying in spaces that keep you small hurts more. It's not failure – try reframing it as protecting your peace and creating space for the kind of support you genuinely need.

Recognizing a toxic relationship

Toxic relationships often drain your energy and self-esteem rather than support and uplift you. They may involve constant criticism, manipulation, or a lack of empathy for your struggles. Gaslighting – where your feelings and experiences are dismissed or twisted to make you doubt yourself – can also be a hallmark of these relationships. You might feel like you're always walking on eggshells, afraid of expressing your true feelings or boundaries. This fear can be especially strong in group situations, where speaking up or being honest about what's on your mind feels even more daunting. In these relationships, your worth is often continually questioned, and rather than feeling seen and understood, you feel diminished or dismissed.

If you have a heavy mental burden, recognizing toxic dynamics can be even more challenging. Feelings of unworthiness, or the belief that you don't deserve better, can keep you tethered to people who reinforce negative feelings about yourself. It becomes particularly difficult when the group engages in behaviours that no longer align with your healing process – such as substance use, unhealthy dieting habits, or taking steroids – and when your efforts to change unsettle them. As you grow and begin to prioritize your healing, not everyone will be supportive of these changes. Some people may struggle with their own unresolved issues, and your progress might highlight what they haven't addressed in themselves. This can create tension in your relationships, making it harder to distance yourself from those who are uncomfortable with your growth or who may subtly (or overtly) try to hold you back. It's difficult when the people you care about become resistant to the healthier path you're choosing, but recognizing these dynamics is an important part of moving forward.

Why letting go is so hard

The fear of loneliness, or the belief that you won't find healthier, more supportive relationships, can also make it difficult to let go. Letting go can feel almost impossible, particularly when you have convinced yourself that you don't deserve more. You might cling to these connections, even when they harm you, because they feel familiar or because you fear that ending them will leave you isolated. Toxic relationships often feed your insecurities, making it harder to walk away.

However, you can't heal in places where you've been hurt. This applies not only to romantic and sexual relationships but to friendships and family connections as well. If someone in your life consistently makes you feel less than, undervalued, or unsafe, it's time to reconsider the role they play in your journey to healing.

The emotional impact of leaving

Leaving a toxic relationship is rarely straightforward. Even if you know it's the right decision, it can be emotionally devastating to let go of someone who has been a significant part of your life. Allow yourself to grieve for these relationships fully rather than intellectualizing the process. You may feel a deep sense of loss, and that's normal – just because a relationship is harmful doesn't mean there weren't moments of connection or love. It's essential to feel the emotions of separation rather than trying to rationalize them away.

Seeing the ending of these relationships as a step towards wholeness rather than focusing on the sense of failure or finality can help reframe the experience. You aren't cutting ties as an act of resentment but to create space for healthier, more supportive connections. Grieving the loss, while difficult, is part of moving forward and making room for relationships that encourage growth and healing. It's also important to let go of worrying about what others may think of your decision. You won't be able to please everyone, and some may not understand why you need to step away. This is where digging deep and trusting yourself becomes an integral part of this process. A therapist or professional can help guide you through this process, offering support as you navigate the emotional challenges of letting go and reinforcing that your healing must come first.

Navigating social media

Social media is quite complex to navigate. While it offers the potential for connection and support, it can also become a source of stress and triggers, particularly when it comes to body image. If you're finding that social media is affecting how you view your body or your mental health, it might be time to take a step back and evaluate how you engage with it.

How is social media making you feel?

The first step in managing the impact of social media is to assess how it's affecting you. Ask yourself: how do you feel after scrolling through your feeds? Do certain posts make you feel more insecure about your body or amplify your feelings of inadequacy? Common triggers could be influencers, fitness accounts, thirst traps – those posts meant to highlight someone's physical appeal, or even well-meaning friends who frequently post about weight loss or appearance. Keep in mind that what you see online is often a heavily filtered version of reality. The people you follow might not intend to cause harm, but their content can still drive unhealthy comparisons.

It's also important to remember that social media is a numbers game, designed to trigger emotional responses, capture attention, and keep you engaged. The platforms are built around algorithms that amplify content that provokes reactions, meaning that what you see isn't just curated by the people you follow but by systems designed to keep you scrolling. Recognizing this can help you step back and make more mindful choices about what content you consume.

Strategies for curating your social media for mental health

You have control over what you see on social media. Curating your feed to promote a healthier mindset is an essential part of protecting your mental well-being.

- Edit your 'for you' page: Take time to examine your feed. Is the content you're consuming making you feel uplifted or more anxious? Consider editing your feed to include more body-positive accounts or following people who promote self-love and diversity in body shapes. You can also use 'not interested', 'mute', or 'unfollow' options for people whose content triggers negative emotions without causing any social discomfort.
- Assess your own social media presence: Don't just focus on the people you follow – think about what you're posting too. Are you contributing to the comparison game? Are you putting pressure on yourself to present a certain image or even to post regularly just to keep up appearances? Reflecting on your own social media presence can be just as important as curating your feed.
- Follow positive influencers: Seek out communities and influencers that encourage authenticity, body neutrality, and kindness. These spaces can counterbalance appearance-focused content and remind you that everyone's journey is unique.

Using social media to find supportive communities

While social media can be a minefield for comparison and self-criticism, it also offers spaces where solidarity and support thrive. There are many communities – particularly within LGBTQ+ spaces – that focus on body positivity, self-acceptance, and mental health. Joining these communities can provide a much-needed sense of belonging and remind you that you're not alone in your struggles. Look for body-positive hashtags or accounts that discuss mental health in an honest and open way. Whether it's a forum, a Facebook group, or an Instagram community, connecting with others who understand your experiences and feel a breath of fresh air provides support and a sense of belonging.

Hookup apps

Hookup apps can be both a source of connection and a potential trigger for body image issues. These apps, with their emphasis on physical appearance, measurements, and body type stats, can often exacerbate feelings of comparison and inadequacy, as users are constantly confronted with curated images of others. If you're finding that these apps are making you feel worse about yourself, it might be worth considering a break or re-evaluating your relationship with them.

Additionally, these apps can become spaces for behaviours that may trigger you, such as 'party and play' (PnP) or 'high and horny' (HnH) culture, where substance use is tied to sexual encounters. For those in recovery or who are triggered by these behaviours, the environment can feel overwhelming and toxic.

The dismissive behaviour often found on these apps can also be damaging. It's not uncommon to encounter rudeness, ghosting, or even being blocked after sending a picture. This kind of rejection, especially when it feels impersonal or transactional, can deeply impact your self-esteem, leaving you feeling devalued and insecure. It can also reinforce the impression that we expect modern-day dating to be this way – detached, quick, and lacking in genuine connection.

Is it time to take a break?

Ask yourself what you're really getting from these apps. Are they fulfilling your need for connection, or are they fuelling the comparability process, making you feel more insecure? If you find that using these apps is triggering, it may be time to take a break. Remember, stepping away doesn't mean you're missing out; it's about prioritizing your mental health and protecting your healing space.

Explore healthy alternatives

Apps that focus on friendship, community-building, or shared interests may provide a more meaningful way to connect without the heavy focus on physical appearance. Platforms like Meetup, local LGBTQ+ groups, or even dating apps that prioritize deeper connections can offer more supportive environments for emotional well-being.

What's missing when you give them up?

One of the hardest aspects of stepping away from hookup apps is dealing with the sense that you're missing out. These apps are often framed as quick ways to find validation or connection, but it's worth asking what is really missing when you give them up? Is it truly connection, or is it the rush of validation? While the initial boost from a match or a conversation can feel good, the long-term emotional toll may outweigh the benefits if the process leaves you feeling worse about yourself. Taking a step back can offer clarity, allowing you to focus on relationships and interactions that truly nurture you rather than ones that reinforce negative self-perceptions.

Ultimately, how you engage with social media and apps is within your control. You have the power to curate your digital experience, edit what you consume, and make choices that serve your mental health. This might mean muting accounts, taking breaks from certain platforms, or even leaving spaces that no longer feel supportive. The goal isn't to disconnect from the world but to connect in healthier, more meaningful ways.

Letting go of the pressure to be constantly present on social media or hookup apps can feel liberating. Taking control of your digital environment protects your mental well-being and creates space for healthier relationships – with others and with yourself.

Relationships and intimacy

Intimacy is difficult for many of us, particularly for gay individuals. When you add the extra layer of body dysmorphia, it can make intimate relationships feel even more complex, personal, and often nerve-wracking. Romantic relationships are often grounded in physical attraction, and emotional closeness can stir up feelings of insecurity, shame, fear, and doubt about whether you're truly deserving of love. It can feel like a recipe for anxiety, with key ingredients including the fear of being assessed on an attractiveness scale, feeling external pressures of what relationships should look like, old traumas resurfacing, and the vulnerability of opening yourself up to someone.

The difficulty of accepting love

One of the most challenging aspects of navigating intimate relationships with body dysmorphia is allowing yourself to believe that you are worthy of love. When you hold negative perceptions of your body, it's easy to feel like your partner's affection or desire for you is misplaced. You may even unconsciously believe that your partner sees you in the same way you see yourself, leading you to doubt their intentions and question how they could possibly be attracted to you or be truly in love with you. This deepens feelings of inadequacy and can create distance in the relationship as you wrestle internally with whether you truly deserve the love being offered.

You may start questioning whether you need to change or improve yourself to be worthy of your partner's affection. For instance, do you find yourself exercising or grooming more, not for your own well-being but to meet what you think are your partner's expectations? It's a fine line between taking care of yourself for confidence and doing it out of fear that you're not attractive enough for someone else. This can often happen in the early stages, before you feel comfortable enough to relax and be yourself.

Additionally, the perfectionist mindset that often accompanies body dysmorphia can spill over into relationships, where you may expect everything to go smoothly or feel pressure for the relationship to be flawless. At the first sign of conflict or imperfection – whether it's a disagreement or a perceived slight – you might be tempted to throw the relationship away or distance yourself, convinced that it's doomed to fail. This hyper-vigilance can cause you to interpret normal relationship challenges as insurmountable, leading to an overly quick retreat rather than working through the issues constructively. It's important to remember that relationships, like people, aren't perfect, and learning to navigate these hurdles is key to building lasting connections.

When new connections spark old patterns

Meeting someone new while dealing with body dysmorphia can feel overwhelming, especially if both of you bring histories of trauma, intimacy issues, and coping mechanisms. In these early encounters, insecurities about appearance can overshadow genuine connection. You might find yourself caught in a cycle of self-critique, focusing on flaws rather than staying present. Old patterns from past relationships may surface, making it easy to fall into an almost automatic assessment – comparing and sizing each other up rather than engaging openly.

These feelings can prompt the urge to 'improve' yourself, thinking it will make you more desirable. However, this often comes from a place of insecurity rather than genuine self-care. Ironically, your partner may already appreciate you as you are, free from the critical lens you apply to yourself. The real challenge, therefore, lies in easing this self-critique, allowing you to stay engaged and be seen as you are.

In these moments, avoiding the temptation to take flight at the first sign of discomfort is vital. These early relationship challenges can actually offer valuable insights if approached mindfully. Instead of shutting down or defaulting to self-critical habits, try to acknowledge what's bubbling up within you. Stay with the discomfort, much like holding a strong yoga pose – breathing through it, even when it feels awkward. This is an opportunity to get curious about your feelings, learning not to run from them or judge yourself harshly. Over time, this practice can help you stay present during moments of vulnerability, welcoming the ebb and flow of intimacy without needing things to be perfect.

Shared insecurities

Your partner may also be dealing with their own self-confidence and intimacy issues. Just as you might feel the pressure to look or act a certain way, they could be struggling with similar insecurities. Recognizing that both of you may be navigating these challenges can create a space for empathy and mutual support. Open communication about these feelings can help both of you find comfort in each other's vulnerability, rather than masking insecurities or striving for unattainable ideals.

The fear of being fully seen

While falling in love can often feel easy, allowing someone to see and accept you fully – imperfections and all – is much harder, especially when body image issues are at play. The initial rush of infatuation might feel exhilarating, but letting someone see you for who you truly are can stir up fears of abandonment, rejection, and judgement.

Moving forward requires becoming more aware of your thoughts and behaviours and challenging the fear of vulnerability that often accompanies intimacy. Intimacy isn't just about physical closeness; it's being emotionally open and accepting that love is rooted in who you are as a person, not just in how you look. Letting go of the belief that you need to 'earn' love through a certain appearance allows you to open yourself up to a more authentic, meaningful relationship – one built on trust, emotional depth, and mutual respect. Only by embracing this mindset can you break down the walls that body dysmorphia may have built, enabling a deeper connection that is based on who you are, not how you look.

Navigating sex with body dysmorphia

Sex is an area where insecurities about our bodies are magnified. Insecurities don't just linger in the background – they can dominate your thoughts and feelings in ways that make intimacy difficult, even painful. The act of being physically exposed, of allowing someone else to see and touch your bare body, can feel like standing under a harsh spotlight. Instead of sex being relaxed and a source of connection or pleasure, it can become a space filled with anxiety, self-doubt, and shame.

There can be immense pressure to engage in sexual relationships even when you're struggling with your self-image. You might feel like you should be having sex or feel like you need to 'perform' sexually to fit into a standard you don't feel capable of reaching. This can make it truly hard to connect with someone intimately. The focus shifts away from connection and towards ticking off boxes in an attempt to avoid rejection. Intimacy becomes something to endure rather than a moment of closeness and pleasure.

When you're in this headspace, it's hard to be present with your partner. Instead of enjoying the moment, you might be consumed by thoughts like, *What are they noticing about my body? Are they seeing the flaws I obsess over? Will they lose interest once they really see me?* For some, past sexual trauma may also resurface, adding another layer of emotional complexity. These fears can lead to dissociation – mentally checking out during sex because you don't feel safe. You might find yourself zoning out, focusing on the performance of sex rather than the experience, just waiting for it to be over so you can finally relax. While dissociation might feel like a way to protect yourself, it stops you from fully engaging in the intimacy and can make the experience feel even more isolating.

Using alcohol or substances

For some people, alcohol or drugs seem like a way to ease the anxiety that comes with sex. It might feel easier to lower your guard and quiet your insecurities after a few drinks or while under the influence. But while these substances can temporarily reduce inhibitions, they also disconnect you from the experience, making it harder to be present with your partner.

Relying on alcohol or drugs to manage intimacy can create a cycle where you feel dependent on them to engage in sex. This emotional distance can make true connection more difficult and, over time, deepen feelings of inadequacy. Learning to navigate intimacy while sober allows for more genuine connections, where you can feel truly accepted for who you are – not just as someone hiding behind a temporary escape.

Relieve the pressure

Sex on your terms is paramount. This might involve communicating your vulnerabilities with a partner or taking time to focus on healing. These steps may feel unconventional, but it's vital that you listen to your own needs rather than external pressures. The goal is to create an environment where your emotional and physical safety are prioritized, even if that means slowing things down or pausing intimacy entirely.

This also means being able to say no. If something doesn't feel right – whether it's not feeling a connection with someone or being uncomfortable with a particular sexual activity – you have the right to stop. Trusting your instincts is an important act of self-respect. Your body is yours, and you are in control of who you share it with, when, and how. A partner who values you will respect your boundaries and understand that true intimacy is built on mutual trust and comfort.

Building confidence in sexual relationships

Building confidence in intimacy isn't about achieving a perfect body or reaching a set standard. It's about learning to accept where you are right now, imperfections and all. Confidence comes from realizing that your worth isn't tied to how you look but to who you are.

Start by paying attention to your thoughts and behaviours surrounding intimate moments. Do you find yourself obsessing over how you look during sex rather than how it feels? Do you avoid certain positions or lighting to hide perceived flaws? While it's natural to have preferences, it's important to ask whether these behaviours are driven by insecurity. It's a gentle reminder that your partner is with you because they're attracted to you as a whole person, not just your body.

It can also help to focus on what makes you feel emotionally safe during intimacy. This might mean starting with affectionate, non-sexual moments like cuddling or holding hands, before diving into more intimate experiences. If you're planning a hookup, consider meeting for coffee or spending time together beforehand to gauge the connection. Confidence grows when you feel secure – both in yourself and in the relationship. As you become more comfortable with vulnerability, intimacy becomes less about appearance and more about shared connection.

Reclaiming intimacy on your terms

Sex, particularly when you're dealing with body dysmorphia, can feel overwhelming. But it's possible to reclaim intimacy on your own terms. This might mean stepping back from sexual relationships for a while to focus on your healing or slowly rebuilding intimacy with a trusted partner. There's no rush and no right way to navigate this journey; what matters is that you feel safe and empowered every step of the way.

Intimacy isn't a race, and there's no one-size-fits-all approach to what it should look like. The goal is to feel emotionally and physically safe, to trust that your worth is not tied to your appearance, and to embrace the idea that true intimacy comes from being seen as a whole person, not just a body.

An evolving support system

As your healing journey continues, so too will your relationships – both personal and romantic. As you evolve, your connections with others will naturally change. Some relationships may deepen as you grow more comfortable with vulnerability, while others may no longer serve the healthier version of yourself that you are becoming. This evolution is a natural part of the process and an opportunity to align yourself with people who truly support and uplift you.

It's important to actively nurture your support system. Your needs today might not be the same in a year, and your circle of support should reflect those changes. Stay open to forming new connections – whether through friendships, communities, or intimate relationships – that help reinforce your self-worth. Surround yourself with people who see you for more than just your appearance and who value your emotional and personal growth.

At the heart of this journey is the understanding that you deserve relationships where you feel safe to be yourself – without a mask, without hiding. You deserve connections that embrace you fully, where your vulnerabilities are met with compassion, and where your growth is not only supported but celebrated. Keep seeking out those who uplift you, and as you continue to heal, remember that you are worthy of love and support, exactly as you are.

CHAPTER 10

Embracing a Reconstructed Identity

As we bring this book to a close, I want to offer a gentle reminder: healing from body dysmorphia is not a straight path. It is continuous, evolving, and deeply personal. The road to self-acceptance and mental wellness is full of highs and lows, breakthroughs and setbacks. Through it all, resilience is born – not as something magical or innate but as a skill cultivated with time, patience, and unwavering commitment to self-love.

Think of this journey like the Japanese art of kintsugi, where broken pottery is mended with gold, making it even more beautiful and unique than before. Healing doesn't erase our cracks and struggles; rather, it highlights them with resilience, turning them into something precious, reflecting our past woven into our identity.

The gay lived experience, and particularly the pressure to conform or look a certain way, can feel relentless. But it's in these moments of relentless pressure that we find the strength to push back, redefine ourselves, and live more authentically. By now, you've likely realized that well-being isn't about perfecting your body, nailing the perfect workout, or following the most rigorous diet plan. It's about reshaping how you see yourself. It's about releasing those external expectations and recognizing the inherent worth you carry within, no matter what your physical appearance may be. True empowerment lies in this shift, in letting go of those burdens and embracing the freedom that comes from knowing you are enough.

Healing means cultivating a compassionate dialogue with yourself, replacing harsh self-criticism with understanding and kindness. The mirror may always be there, but it doesn't have to define you. You are more than your reflection – you are your thoughts, your dreams, your creativity, your relationships, and your impact on the world around you. To embrace this broader sense of identity is to start living beyond dysmorphia.

As you heal, take note of any self-sabotage that may arise. Sometimes you may feel drawn to return to old habits or behaviours, especially when facing discomfort. It's natural to seek what feels familiar, even if it doesn't serve you. For example, you might find yourself slipping back into critical self-talk or restrictive routines because they feel 'safe'. Recognizing these moments with compassion is key; they're signals that healing is moving you out of your comfort zone. Remember, your journal is your friend here; use it to express your thoughts and help you make connections.

Empowering your true self

As you've journeyed through these chapters, you've likely come to realize that true empowerment comes from accepting who you are, flaws and all. Healing is reconnecting with who you've always been, buried under the layers of doubt and societal expectations. It's about peeling back those layers to reveal a self that is whole, worthy, and deserving of love.

Building an identity grounded in acceptance requires daily practice. Just as neurones in our brain wire together through repeated thought patterns, so too must our self-talk and behaviours reflect this shift. 'Neurones that fire together, wire together' – meaning, the more we practise self-love, the more natural it becomes. It takes effort to turn the tide against years of self-criticism, but with each step forward, you move closer to embodying your empowered, authentic self.

Embracing the hard days

I want you to know that there will still be off days – days where the old thoughts creep in, where the mirror catches your eye, and those familiar feelings of inadequacy bubble to the surface. But these days are not setbacks; they are a normal part of the journey. Learning to accept and welcome these feelings is essential. Healing doesn't mean never feeling bad again. It means allowing yourself to sit with whatever emotion arises rather than fleeing from it.

When these moments arise, pause. Breathe. Ask yourself: what does my body, my heart need right now? This could be rest, nourishment, or even a conversation with someone who loves you. Trust your intuition in these moments and listen closely to what your inner voice is telling you. Off days are not the end of your journey; they are opportunities to practise the self-compassion you've been cultivating. If you need guidance, I invite you to return to some of the exercises throughout this book, which may help ground you in the moment.

Healing hurts - but it's worth it

Healing is one of the most painful yet beautiful things you can do for yourself. It brings to the surface emotions you've buried, traumas you've locked away, and vulnerabilities you've guarded fiercely. But as you dig through these layers, you uncover strength, wisdom, and a deeper understanding of who you are.

This process requires not just confronting your pain but working through it. You are your healer. No one can do it for you. No therapist, friend, or partner can resolve the deep-rooted beliefs you hold about yourself. They can support and guide you, but the power to heal rests with you. You are the architect of your mental wellness, and you have everything within you to rebuild from the inside out.

The new relationship with yourself

As you heal, you are entering into a new relationship – with yourself. You're falling in love with who you are, not as an idea but as a whole, imperfect person. Date yourself. Nourish yourself. Invest in yourself. Every moment spent cultivating self-love is a step towards building the kind of relationship with yourself that no external validation can provide. This relationship won't always be easy. Like all relationships, it requires effort, patience, boundaries, and understanding. Keep showing up for yourself. Keep believing in yourself, even when it feels like no one else does.

In this new relationship, be cautious of meta-addictions – the tendency to become addicted to self-improvement itself, feeling compelled to constantly 'fix' every aspect of your being. Meta-addictions can show up as an endless cycle of self-help books, healing retreats, and daily mental checklists, all creating the illusion of progress while keeping you in a loop of never feeling 'enough'. Sound familiar?! In recent years, trauma has become a buzzword, often associated with various health trends. While it's important to address our past, it's also important not to let it define our every waking moment. The key is to find balance; healing is essential, but sometimes the most healing thing you can do is be in the present moment, detached from the need to improve, and simply live life beyond your wounds, embracing the freedom that comes from just *being* and not thinking too much.

Final words: a commitment to self-love

The privilege of a lifetime is to become who you truly are. As you move forward on this journey, focus on choosing compassion over self-criticism. Even on difficult days, when believing in yourself feels hard, commit to it anyway. Remember, certainty is an illusion – life will always be filled with unknowns, and that's okay. Learning to swim in uncertainty is part of growth. Above all, your inner world is your priority. The love you nurture within yourself will form the foundation for all your other relationships. When you cultivate this inner love, it radiates outward and shapes how you connect with others.

This book has been my healing journey. Each chapter is a reflection of the lessons I've learnt, the struggles I've faced, and the victories I've celebrated. But now it's your journey. Take these words, these insights, and apply them to your life in a way that feels right for you. There's no rush, no finish line – just a steady commitment to loving yourself exactly as you are.

As you continue on this path, know that you are not alone. Your journey matters, and you deserve all the love, peace, and acceptance this world has to offer. If this book has resonated with you, I encourage you to stay connected by joining my community, where we can continue this conversation, support one another, and celebrate our growth together. You don't have to face this journey in isolation – there are people out there who understand and will walk with you.

https://danieloshaughnessy.com/linktree

With this final reflection, the book comes to a close, but your story continues. *You are the author now.*

Final exercise: Reconnecting with your younger self

In this final reflection, I encourage you to reconnect with your younger self – the version of you who first began struggling with body image before you had the tools or understanding to navigate those feelings. This practice is about offering compassion and love to that younger version of yourself who may have felt lost, misunderstood, or inadequate. It's a chance to heal the past and, in doing so, build a stronger foundation for the future.

Find a quiet space where you can sit without distractions. Close your eyes and take a few deep breaths, feeling the air fill your lungs and release. With each breath, allow yourself to relax deeper into the moment, letting go of any tension in your body or mind.

Now, picture yourself walking through a peaceful, open space – perhaps a field, a beach, or a quiet park. As you walk, you notice a figure in the distance. As you get closer, you realize it's your younger self, from the time when body dysmorphia first started shaping how you saw yourself. You can see in their eyes the uncertainty, the confusion, maybe even the pain. You know these feelings all too well because you've carried them with you for years.

Approach your younger self gently, as if greeting an old friend. Sit with them – maybe on a bench or a soft patch of grass. Look into their eyes, and when you're ready, start a conversation. What would you like to say? This is your chance to offer them the words you needed to hear at that time. Perhaps you'll remind them that they are beautiful, just as they are. Maybe you'll reassure them that it's okay to feel vulnerable and that their worth is not tied to how they look.

Now take a moment to listen. What does your younger self want to say to you? What do they need to feel safe, supported, and understood? Allow them to express their fears and insecurities without judgement. You may feel emotions welling up as you listen – let yourself feel them fully. This is part of the healing process.

As you both sit together in this peaceful space, offer your younger self a gesture of love. It might be a hug, a smile, or simply holding their hand. Let them know they are not alone and that they never were. Reassure them that their struggles were valid, but that they have grown stronger through every challenge. You are here for them now, with all the wisdom, compassion, and love you've gained along the way.

Before you say goodbye, remind your younger self that the journey ahead won't always be easy. There will still be trials and tribulations – moments of doubt, days where the old thoughts resurface – but they are resilient, and so are you. Healing can be bumpy with ups and downs. Let your younger self know that no matter how difficult it may feel at times, they must never give up. The love, peace, and self-acceptance they seek are worth the effort.

As you stand up and prepare to leave, thank your younger self for everything they have taught you – about strength, vulnerability, and resilience. Know that this connection is not lost. You can return to this space at any time to offer them comfort and reassurance. Carry this healing with you as you walk back towards the present moment, feeling a deeper sense of peace and compassion for who you were, who you are, and who you are becoming.

When you are ready, gently open your eyes and take a few deep breaths, carrying the love and wisdom of this reflection with you.

Resources

Body dysmorphia specific support

- Body Dysmorphic Disorder Foundation is a UK-based charity offering support for individuals struggling with body dysmorphic disorder. https://bddfoundation.org
- International OCD Foundation, based in the United States, focuses on obsessive-compulsive disorder and related disorders, including body dysmorphia. They provide resources for individuals worldwide. https://iocdf.org

LGBTQ+ support

- Switchboard is a confidential listening service for the LGBTQ+ communities. https://switchboard.lgbt
- Stonewall campaigns for the equality of lesbian, gay, bi, and trans people across Britain. www.stonewall.org.uk
- LGBT Foundation is a national charity delivering advice, support, and information services to LGBTQ+ communities. https://lgbt.foundation
- LGBT Health and Wellbeing works to improve the health, well-being and equality of LGBTQ+ people in Scotland. www.lgbthealth.org.uk
- LGBT Cymru Helpline offers support and information to the LGBTQ+ community in Wales. www.lgbtcymru.org.uk
- You Are Loved CIC is a UK-based, queer-led nonprofit organization dedicated to reducing deaths from suicide and

drug-related causes among LGBTQ+ individuals. www.youare-loved.com

International LGBTQ+ support

- Egale Canada works to improve the lives of LGBTQ+ people in Canada and offers resources for mental health, legal support, and general well-being. https://egale.ca
- Gay Helpline is an Italian organization offering support services to the LGBTQ+ community, with helplines in Italian and English. https://gayhelpline.it
- International Lesbian, Gay, Bisexual, Trans, and Intersex Association is a global organization that advocates for LGBTQ+ rights and provides resources and support across many countries. https://ilga.org
- OutRight Action International advocates for the rights of LGBTQ+ people globally and works to prevent persecution and discrimination. It offers resources and support for international communities. https://outrightinternational.org
- Rainbow Railroad helps LGBTQ+ individuals escape persecution and violence in countries where it is unsafe to live openly. www.rainbowrailroad.org
- It Gets Better Project offers encouragement and support to LGBTQ+ youth by sharing stories of overcoming adversity and creating hope. https://itgetsbetter.org
- Trevor Project, based in the United States, offers crisis intervention and suicide prevention services for LGBTQ+ youth and provides global resources for mental health and well-being. www.thetrevorproject.org

Drugs and alcohol

- Antidote at London Friend is one of the UK's only LGBTQ+ run and targeted drug and alcohol support networks. https://londonfriend.org.uk

Nationwide 12-step groups

A 12-step programme is a set of guiding principles outlining a course of action for recovery from addiction, compulsion, or other behavioural problems. Some have specific LGBTQ+ meetings, so look at what your local meeting provides.

- Alcoholics Anonymous: www.alcoholics-anonymous.org.uk
- Cocaine Anonymous: www.cocaineanonymous.org.uk
- Crystal Meth Anonymous: www.crystalmeth.org.uk
- Narcotics Anonymous: https://ukna.org

International 12-step groups

For individuals outside the UK, here are the international websites for the key 12-step programmes:

- Alcoholics Anonymous: www.aa.org
- Narcotics Anonymous: www.na.org

Sexual health and HIV

- 56 Dean Street is a friendly, convenient, and free NHS sexual health clinic in the heart of London. The Soho-based service also offers full outpatient HIV clinic services. www.dean.st
- Gay Men Fighting AIDS is a gay men's health and sexual health project. www.gmfa.org.uk
- Terrence Higgins Trust is a national HIV and sexual health charity with information on HIV, sexually transmitted infections, and where to get tested. www.tht.org.uk
- Positively UK can support any aspect of your diagnosis, care, and living with HIV. https://positivelyuk.org

Therapy

The following are databases to seek help from a qualified therapist. Ensure that the therapist you choose understands LGBTQ+ issues.

- British Association for Counselling and Psychotherapy: www.bacp.co.uk
- Pink Therapy: directory of LGBTQ+ therapists: www.pinktherapy.com
- UK Council for Psychotherapy: www.psychotherapy.org.uk

Mental health

- Beat Eating Disorders is a directory of support services and information targeted at those with eating disorders. www.beateatingdisorders.org.uk
- Mind gives information about mental health support. www.mind.org.uk
- Mind Out is a mental health service run by and for LGBTQ+ people with experience of mental health issues. www.mindout.org.uk
- Samaritans offers a safe place for you to talk about whatever is on your mind. Call free on 116 123 at any time. www.samaritans.org

Trauma and mental health

- PTSD UK provides support for those dealing with post-traumatic stress disorder, which can be relevant to individuals experiencing trauma-related issues. www.ptsduk.org
- Trauma Foundation provides global resources and support for trauma recovery, focusing on education and therapy for those impacted by trauma. https://thetraumafoundation.org

Housing

- Albert Kennedy Trust helps young LGBTQ+ people who are made homeless or living in a hostile environment by providing housing and services to help them live independently. www.akt.org.uk

References

Bhasin, S., Brito, J.P., Cunningham, G.R., Hayes, F.J. *et al.* (2018) 'Testosterone therapy in men with hypogonadism: An Endocrine Society clinical practice guideline.' *Journal of Clinical Endocrinology & Metabolism 10, 35,* 1–36. https://doi.org/10.1210/jc.2018-01629

Bremner, J.D. (2006) 'Traumatic stress: Effects on the brain.' *Dialogues in Clinical Neuroscience 8, 4,* 445–461.

Chakrabarti, A., Geurts, L., Hoyles, L., Iozzo, P. *et al.* (2022) 'The microbiota–gut–brain axis: Pathways to better brain health. Perspectives on what we know, what we need to investigate and how to put knowledge into practice.' *Cellular and Molecular Life Sciences 79, 2,* 80.

Chekroud, S.R., Gueorguieva, R., Zheutlin, A.B., Paulus, M. *et al.* (2018) 'Association between physical exercise and mental health in 1.2 million individuals in the USA between 2011 and 2015: A cross-sectional study.' *The Lancet Psychiatry 5, 9,* 739–746. https://doi.org/10.1016/S2215-0366(18)30227-X

Cohen, B.E., Edmondson, D., and Kronish, I.M. (2015) 'State of the art review: Depression, stress, anxiety, and cardiovascular disease.' *American Journal of Hypertension 28, 11,* 1295–1302.

Didie, E.R., Menard, W., Stern, A.P., and Phillips, K.A. (2008) 'Occupational functioning and impairment in adults with body dysmorphic disorder.' *Comprehensive Psychiatry 49, 6,* 561–569.

Downs, A. (2012) *The Velvet Rage: Overcoming the Pain of Growing Up Gay in a Straight Man's World* (rev. ed.). Da Capo Press.

Edwards, C., Havlik, J., Cong, W., Mullen, W. *et al.* (2017) 'Polyphenols and health: Interactions between fibre, plant polyphenols and the gut microbiota.' *Nutrition Bulletin, 42,* 356–360. https://doi.org/10.1111/nbu.12296

Filice, E., Raffoul, A., Meyer, S.B., and Neiterman, E. (2020) 'The impact of social media on body image perceptions and bodily practices among gay, bisexual, and other men who have sex with men: A critical review of the literature and extension of theory.' *Sex Roles, 82,* 387–410.

Firth, J., Gangwisch, J.E., Borsini, A., Wootton, R.E., and Mayer, E.A. (2020) 'Food and mood: How do diet and nutrition affect mental wellbeing? *BMJ 369,* m2382. https://doi.org/10.1136/bmj.m2382

Glaser, R. and Kiecolt-Glaser, J.K. (2005) 'Stress-induced immune dysfunction: Implications for health.' *Nature Reviews Immunology 5, 3,* 243–251.

Grajek, M., Krupa-Kotara, K., Białek-Dratwa, A., Sobczyk, K. *et al.* (2022) 'Nutrition and mental health: A review of current knowledge about the impact of diet on mental health.' *Frontiers in Nutrition* 9, 943998.

Griffin, B.J., Worthington, E.L., Lavelock, C.R., Wade, N.G., and Hoyt, W.T. (2015) 'Forgiveness and Mental Health.' In L. Toussaint, E. Worthington, and D. Williams (eds), *Forgiveness and Health: Scientific Evidence and Theories Relating Forgiveness to Better Health.* Springer. https://doi.org/10.1007/978-94-017-9993-5_6

Griffiths, S., Murray, S.B., Krug, I., and McLean, S.A. (2018) 'The contribution of social media to body dissatisfaction, eating disorder symptoms, and anabolic steroid use among sexual minority men.' *Cyberpsychology, Behavior, and Social Networking, 21,* 3, 149–156. https://doi.org/10.1089/cyber.2017.0375

Hackett, G., Kirby, M., Rees, R.W., Jones, T.H. *et al.* (2023) 'The British Society for Sexual Medicine guidelines on male adult testosterone deficiency, with statements for practice.' *World Journal of Men's Health 41,* 3, 508–537. https://doi.org/10.5534/wjmh.221027

Hausenblas, H.A. and Fallon, E.A. (2006) 'Exercise and body image: A meta-analysis.' *Psychology & Health 21,* 1, 33–47. https://doi.org/10.1080/14768320500105270

Kessler, R.C., Sonnega, A., Bromet, E., Hughes, M., and Nelson, C.B. (2013) 'Post-traumatic Stress Disorder in the National Comorbidity Survey.' In S. Hyman (ed.), *Fear and Anxiety.* Routledge.

Kutscher, E., Arshed, A., Greene, R.E., and Kladney, M. (2024) 'Exploring anabolic androgenic steroid use among cisgender gay, bisexual, and queer men.' *JAMA Network Open, 7,* 5, e2411088–e2411088.

Lawler, K.A., Younger, J.W., Piferi, R.L., Billington, E. *et al.* (2003) 'A change of heart: Cardiovascular correlates of forgiveness in response to interpersonal conflict.' *Journal of Behavioral Medicine 26,* 373–393.

Levin, R.L. and Rawana, J.S. (2016) 'Attention-deficit/hyperactivity disorder and eating disorders across the lifespan: A systematic review of the literature.' *Clinical Psychology Review, 50,* 22–36.

Loucks, E.B., Schuman-Olivier, Z., Saadeh, F.B., Scarpaci, M.M. *et al.* (2023) 'Effect of adapted mindfulness training in participants with elevated office blood pressure: The MB-BP Study: A randomized clinical trial. *Journal of the American Heart Association 12,* 11, e028712. https://doi.org/10.1161/jaha.122.028712

Mahmud, M.R., Akter, S., Tamanna, S.K., Mazumder, L. *et al.* (2022) 'Impact of gut microbiome on skin health: Gut–skin axis observed through the lenses of therapeutics and skin diseases.' *Gut Microbes 14,* 1, 2096995.

Mayer, E.A. (2011) 'Gut feelings: The emerging biology of gut–brain communication.' *Nature Reviews Neuroscience 12,* 8, 453–466. https://doi.org/10.1038/nrn3071

McBeth, J., Morris, S., Benjamin, S., Silman, A.J., and Macfarlane, G. J. (2001) 'Associations between adverse events in childhood and chronic widespread pain in adulthood: Are they explained by differential recall?' *Journal of Rheumatology 28,* 10, 2305–2309.

Mhillaj, E., Morgese, M.G., Tucci, P., Bove, M., Schiavone, S., and Trabace, L. (2015) 'Effects of anabolic-androgens on brain reward function.' *Frontiers in Neuroscience, 9,* 295. https://doi.org/10.3389/fnins.2015.00295

National Health Service (NHS) (2023) *Body dysmorphic disorder (BDD).* www.nhs.uk/mental-health/conditions/body-dysmorphia

Nutt, D., Spriggs, M., and Erritzoe, D. (2023) 'Psychedelics therapeutics: What we know, what we think, and what we need to research.' *Neuropharmacology* 223: 109257.

Office for National Statistics (2023) 'Crime Survey for England and Wales: Drug Misuse Report, 2023.' www.ons.gov.uk/peoplepopulationand-community/crimeandjustice/articles/drugmisuseinenglandandwales/yearendingmarch2023

Oshana, A., Klimek, P., and Blashill, A.J. (2020) 'Minority stress and body dysmorphic disorder symptoms among sexual minority adolescents and adult men.' *Body Image, 34,* 167–174.

O'Shaughnessy, D. (2022) *Naked Nutrition: An LGBTQ+ Guide to Diet and Lifestyle.* Unbound.

Pope Jr, H.G., Kanayama, G., Athey, A., Ryan, E., Hudson, J.I., and Baggish, A. (2014) 'The lifetime prevalence of anabolic androgenic steroid use and dependence in Americans: Current best estimates.' *American Journal on Addictions, 23,* 4, 371–377.

Prichard, I. and Tiggemann, M. (2008) 'Relations among exercise type, self-objectification, and body image in the fitness centre environment: The role of reasons for exercise.' *Psychology of Sport and Exercise 9,* 6, 855–866. https://doi.org/10.1016/j.psychsport.2007.10.005

Radjabzadeh, D., Bosch, J.A., Uitterlinden, A.G., Zwinderman, A.H. *et al.* (2022) 'Gut microbiome-wide association study of depressive symptoms.' *Nature Communications 13,* 1, 7128.

Rosenzweig, S., Greeson, J.M., Reibel, D.K., Green, J.S., Jasser, S.A., and Beasley, D. (2010) 'Mindfulness-based stress reduction for chronic pain conditions: Variation in treatment outcomes and role of home meditation practice.' *Journal of Psychosomatic Research 68,* 1, 29–36.

Rusch, H.L., Rosario, M., Levison, L.M., Olivera, A. *et al.* (2019) 'The effect of mindfulness meditation on sleep quality: A systematic review and meta-analysis of randomized controlled trials.' *Annals of the New York Academy of Sciences 1445,* 1, 5–16. https://doi.org/10.1111/nyas.13996

Sandstrom, G.M. and Dunn, E.W. (2014) 'Is efficiency overrated? Minimal social interactions lead to belonging and positive affect.' *Social Psychological and Personality Science 5,* 4, 437–442.

Schmidt, M., Taube, C.O., Heinrich, T., Vocks, S., and Hartmann, A.S. (2022) 'Body image disturbance and associated eating disorder and body dysmorphic disorder pathology in gay and heterosexual men: A systematic analyses of cognitive, affective, behavioural and perceptual aspects.' *PLOS One, 17,* 12, e0278558.

Shah, J. and Gurbani, S. (2019) 'Association of Vitamin D Deficiency and Mood Disorders: A Systematic Review.' In J. Fedotova (ed.), *Vitamin D Deficiency.* IntechOpen. https://doi.org/10.5772/intechopen.90617

Smith, R.N., Mann, N.J., Braue, A., Mäkeläinen, H., and Varigos, G.A. (2007) 'The effect of a high-protein, low glycemic-load diet versus a conventional, high glycemic-load diet on biochemical parameters associated with acne vulgaris: A randomized, investigator-masked, controlled trial.' *Journal of the American Academy of Dermatology 57*, 2, 247–256. https://doi.org/10.1016/j.jaad.2007.01.046

Tasios, K. and Michopoulos, I. (2017) 'Body dysmorphic disorder: Latest neuroanatomical and neuropsychological findings.' *Psychiatriki, 28*, 3, 242–250.

Tomiyama, A.J., Mann, T., Vinas, D., Hunger, J.M., Dejager, J., and Taylor, S.E. (2010) 'Low calorie dieting increases cortisol.' *Psychosomatic Medicine 72*, 4, 357–364. https://doi.org/10.1097/PSY.0b013e3181d9523c

Valles-Colomer, M., Falony, G., Darzi, Y., Tigchelaar, E. F. *et al.* (2019) 'The neuroactive potential of the human gut microbiota in quality of life and depression.' *Nature Microbiology 4*, 4, 623–632. https://doi.org/10.1038/s41564-018-0337-x

Weiffenbach, A. and Kundu, R.V. (2015) 'Body Dysmorphic Disorder: Etiology and Pathophysiology.' In N.A. Vashi (ed.), *Beauty and Body Dysmorphic Disorder: A Clinician's Guide*. Springer International Publishing.

Wolke, D. and Sapouna, M. (2008) 'Big men feeling small: Childhood bullying experience, muscle dysmorphia and other mental health problems in bodybuilders.' *Psychology of Sport and Exercise, 9*, 5, 595–604.

Yehuda, R., Daskalakis, N.P., Bierer, L.M., Bader, H.N. *et al.* (2016) 'Holocaust exposure induced intergenerational effects on FKBP5 methylation.' *Biological Psychiatry 80*, 5, 372–380. https://doi.org/10.1016/j.biopsych.2015.08.005

Acknowledgements

The process of writing this book has been a whirlwind of healing, one made possible by the extraordinary support of those who stood by me when I needed it most.

To my mother, who believed in my potential every step of the way, cheering me on with unwavering pride. Your love has been my constant guide.

To my dog, Wallis, for softening my heart and teaching me the subtle art of unconditional love. Your presence – patiently waiting under my desk as I write – was, and always is, a balm to my soul.

To the friends who stood by me through the twists and turns of my healing journey and the process of writing this book. For checking in when I needed it most, defending me when I couldn't, and simply being there when I felt lost. Your loyalty has meant the world to me. You each know who you are. This book wouldn't exist without your quiet courage and strength beside me.

To my teachers in life: Dr Miguel Toribio Mateas, who not only served as a rock in my healing journey but also believed in me when I couldn't believe in myself; Professor Brian Sutton, who sparked my creativity and encouraged me to push the boundaries of incorporating the lessons of healing into academic language; Echo Elliot, my yoga teacher, who taught me how to care for, respect, and deeply connect with my body; and Alan Dolan, who generously shared his profound wisdom of breathwork and trained me to become a facilitator. You have each left an indelible mark on my path.

To my therapist, Tiago Brandao, for helping me peel back the layers of shame, trauma, and doubt that once held me captive. Your guidance has been nothing short of life-changing. You've helped me surf the waves of my healing journey, allowing me to make sense of myself and build a new relationship with my body. For that, I am forever grateful.

To Pete Cuthbertson at Sixteen Eleven Consultancy, whose steady PR support has been invaluable in sharing this work with the world. Your expertize made all the difference.

To my agent, Andrew James at Frog Literary, and everyone at Jessica Kingsley Publishers, especially Jane Evans, Sarah Thomson, and Laura Savage – thank you for believing in me and for taking a chance on this book. Your faith in my vision has made it a reality.

To everyone who helped behind the scenes, keeping things running smoothly so I could focus on this work – your support made this possible. A particular thanks to Joshua North and Oksana Yuzhda for making life that bit easier throughout the journey.

To the healers – both seen and unseen – who helped unlock parts of me I never knew existed. You illuminated the path back to myself when I had lost my way.

To my clients and community – thank you for your patience and trust as I went through my own reconstruction. Your belief in me has been both humbling and empowering.

And finally, to my past self. The one who couldn't see a way out. The one who thought hope had long disappeared. Thank you for holding on, for trusting the process, and for being brave enough to keep fighting. This book is the love letter you always deserved.

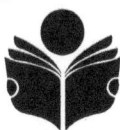

RAISING READERS
Books Build Bright Futures

Dear Reader,

We'd love your attention for one more page to tell you about the crisis in children's reading, and what we can all do.

Studies have shown that reading for fun is the **single biggest predictor of a child's future life chances** – more than family circumstance, parents' educational background or income. It improves academic results, mental health, wealth, communication skills, ambition and happiness.[1]

The number of children reading for fun is in rapid decline. Young people have a lot of competition for their time. In 2024, 1 in 10 children and young people in the UK aged 5 to 18 did not own a single book at home.[2]

Hachette works extensively with schools, libraries and literacy charities, but here are some ways we can all raise more readers:

- Reading to children for just 10 minutes a day makes a difference
- Don't give up if children aren't regular readers – there will be books for them!
- Visit bookshops and libraries to get recommendations
- Encourage them to listen to audiobooks
- Support school libraries
- Give books as gifts

There's a lot more information about how to encourage children to read on our website: **www.RaisingReaders.co.uk**

Thank you for reading.

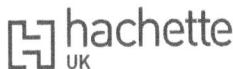

hachette
UK

1   National Literacy Trust, 'Book Ownership in 2024', November 2024, https://literacytrust.org.uk/research-services/research-reports/book-ownership-in-2024
2   OECD, '21st-Century Readers: Developing Literacy Skills in a Digital World', OECD Publishing, Paris, 2021, https://www.oecd.org/en/publications/21st-century-readers_a83d84cb-en.html